A FRAGMENTED FEMINISM

This book is a search for 'the real Anandibai Joshee' – a search in which the readers are invited to participate.

In her short and eventful life, Anandibai Joshee, the first Indian woman to earn a medical degree, broke many stereotypes. Literate at a time when it was taboo for a girl to attend school or even 'pick up a paper', she was courageous, articulate, and assertive. And ambitious. Fuelled by a desire to improve the healthcare that was available to Indian women at that time, she travelled across the seas to the United States to study medicine.

Meera Kosambi's biography of Anandibai is more than just a retelling of the life of a woman who was ahead of her time. Drawing on a host of narratives, Kosambi recovers Anandibai's many voices, which have been submerged in history – that of a conflicted feminist, a nationalist, and a reformer, among others – and her engagement with the world at large.

This book is a testament to Meera Kosambi's commitment to social history. When she passed away in 2015, she left an incomplete manuscript that has been painstakingly put together by the editors. Drawing on archival research, including a host of Anandibai's letters, her poems in Marathi, newspaper reports, and rare photographs, this book will be of immense interest to scholars and researchers of modern Indian history, sociology, gender, and South Asian studies.

The late **Meera Kosambi** was a sociologist who retired as Professor and Director, Research Centre for Women's Studies, Shreemati Nathibai Damodar Thackersey Women's University, Mumbai, Maharashtra, India. She was trained in India, Sweden, and the United States, and specialized in urban studies and women's studies. Her publications include *Gender, Culture and Performance: Marathi Theatre and Cinema before Independence* (2015, Routledge); *Crossing Thresholds* (2007); *Women Writing Gender* (2012); and *Mahatma Gandhi and Prema Kantak* (2013).

Ram Ramaswamy recently retired from the Jawaharlal Nehru University in New Delhi, India, where he had taught in the School of Physical Sciences since 1986. He is presently a visiting professor at the Indian Institute of Technology (IIT)-Delhi. With a sustained interest in the work of Meera Kosambi, and her father D. D. Kosambi, he has, in addition to the present work, edited two collections of D.D. Kosambi's essays and papers, *Adventures into the Unknown: Essays by D. D. Kosambi* (2016) and *D. D. Kosambi: Selected Works in Mathematics and Statistics* (2016).

Madhavi Kolhatkar retired as Professor in Sanskrit Dictionary Project, Deccan College, Pune, India. She has a PhD in Sanskrit from Pune University and working knowledge of German, Russian, Tibetan, and Japanese. She has attended seminars and conferences in the United States, Japan, and Romania; and was invited to Japan for a joint project undertaken by China and Japan. She has authored nine books and more than one hundred articles in English, Sanskrit, and Marathi.

Aban Mukherji is a freelance writer and translator. She has a master's degree in History and has co-translated (with Tulsi Vatsal) *Karan Gehlo*, the first Gujarati novel published in 1866. She has contributed articles to various publications.

A FRAGMENTED FEMINISM

The Life and Letters of Anandibai Joshee

Meera Kosambi

*Edited by Ram Ramaswamy,
Madhavi Kolhatkar,
and Aban Mukherji*

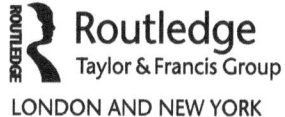

Routledge
Taylor & Francis Group

LONDON AND NEW YORK

First published 2020
by Routledge
2 Park Square, Milton Park, Abingdon, Oxon OX14 4RN

and by Routledge
605 Third Avenue, New York, NY 10017

First issued in paperback 2021

Routledge is an imprint of the Taylor & Francis Group, an informa business

British Library Cataloguing-in-Publication Data
A catalogue record for this book is available from the British Library

Library of Congress Cataloging-in-Publication Data
A catalog record for this book has been requested

Typeset in Garamond
by Apex CoVantage, LLC

ISBN 13: 978-0-367-78412-6 (pbk)
ISBN 13: 978-1-138-38486-6 (hbk)

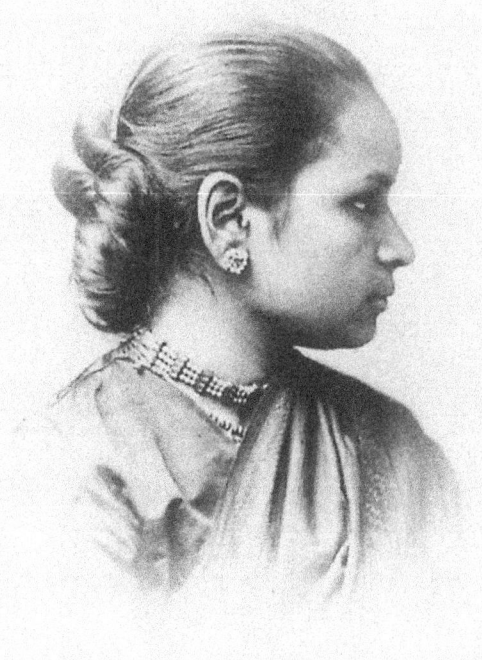

आनंदीबाई जोशी.

Anandibai Joshee

Frontispiece to the 1888 edition of Pandita Ramabai's *The High Caste Hindu Woman*

Source: Wikimedia Commons, courtesy of Legacy Center Archives & Special Collections, Drexel University College of Medicine, Philadelphia. http://drexel.edu/LegacyCenter

CONTENTS

FIGURES

DEDICATION

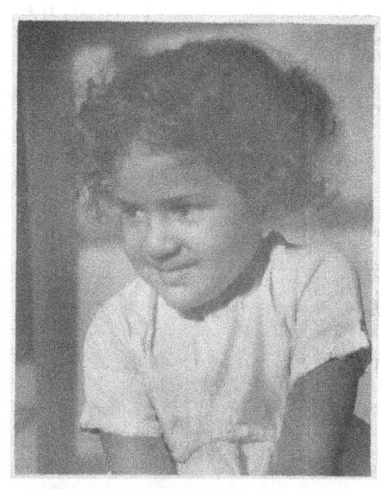

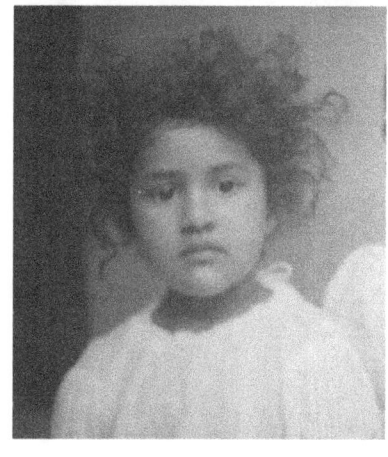

MEERA KOSAMBI (1939–2015)

FOREWORD

Meera Kosambi: friend, scholar, mentor

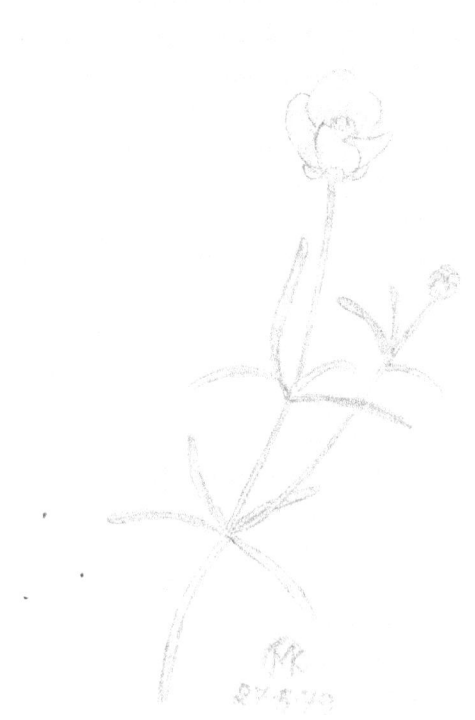

Aban Mukherji: *my friend Meera Kosambi*

It is difficult to write about Meera Kosambi with objectivity and detachment. She entered my life when I was still a schoolgirl in plaits, and soon became part of our family. Vivacious and full of life, she could liven up the dullest gathering. She was like an elder sister to me, encouraging me to do my best and scolding me soundly when I fell short of her expectations.

For many years I took her for granted, as I did my own tolerant and inclusive family. It was only after she became the head of the Research Centre for Women's Studies (RCWS) at the SNDT Women's University[1] and came to live with us in Mumbai for an extended period of time that I began to appreciate her true worth. A 'scholar extraordinaire' she was also, like her father, a polymath in her own right. She was not only a brilliant academic, but also a superb seamstress and embroiderer. She had an eye for fabrics and designed, stitched, and embroidered her own clothes as meticulously as she executed her research work. Moreover, she was an excellent cook and loved trying out new dishes. Her very feminine aesthetic sensibilities could transform the meanest dwelling into a pleasant and warm space. She loved plants and flowers and created a garden wherever she lived.

Meera took up photography with a passion and also loved to paint in her spare time. She was a connoisseur of both Western and Indian classical music and had learnt to sing and play the sitar in her youth. She was an inveterate traveller and had traversed the globe several times.

Meera was fluent in Marathi, English, Hindi, and Swedish and had a fair knowledge of Sanskrit and Pali too. She started out as an urban sociologist and was one of the early scholars who wrote on the development of Mumbai and Pune. She later moved to women's studies and also left her mark on this field. She authored several books on the social history of nineteenth century Maharashtra but died before her magnum opus, *Pandita Ramabai*,[2] could be published. It was her dying wish to see the present work on Anandibai Joshee in print.

Meera's unfinished projects were as remarkable as her completed works. She spent several years on a monumental and taxing project, commissioned by the Census Board, to analyse and assess the various issues relating to women in Maharashtra, spanning a century. Unfortunately, this work could never be brought to fruition, leaving her mentally and physically exhausted, having wasted years of energy on it. Had she completed this work, I personally feel that it would have been one of her greatest contributions as a sociologist.

Meera would often declare that in her old age she would pen a historical novel, a thriller whose plot would be situated in the Medieval

Period. But because of her untimely death from cancer, this project, too, did not see the light of day. Research was Meera's passion, and she could sit for hours in the most uncomfortable places poring over old manuscripts, books, and newspapers, meticulously copying out whole passages in her neat hand. The library of the Asiatic Society became her second home. She would leave our house in the morning to catch the 122 Bus to Ballard Estate, and return dog-tired in the evening, only reviving after innumerable cups of tea.

Her post as director of the RCWS was a demanding one. But with all her gruelling administrative work, she still found time to write numerous books as well as monographs for the Centre. Most of her books were written while she was propped up in bed – all she needed was some peace and quiet, and a steady supply of tea!

Meera also put her heart and soul into mentoring students and the younger staff members, and gave them several opportunities to showcase their talents. But she could be an exacting task master as she refused to settle for anything but the best. If she appeared harsh in her criticism towards others, she was much harder on herself. Living in the shadow of her illustrious father and grandfather, she despaired of ever living up to their standards of excellence. This feeling persisted like a dark cloud over her life, robbing her of any satisfaction she might have felt towards her own work. Her deeply rooted anxiety and lack of self-confidence, though hidden from the world, dogged her all her life and often translated into unreasonable behaviour which unfortunately put off many who might otherwise have befriended her.

Impatient by nature and unable to suffer fools, Meera could be extremely tolerant and understanding towards the people she loved and was ever ready to excuse their shortcomings. She was generous to a fault and would often overwhelm her friends with gifts. For her, friendship went hand in hand with loyalty and self-sacrifice. She totally disregarded her own reputation or well-being when it came to defending or protecting a friend in need of help.

The last few years of Meera's life were lived with a sense of urgency. She knew that she did not have long to live, but she soldiered on alone, determined to keep death at bay for as long as possible. It was a race against time to complete her manuscript on Pandita Ramabai, and she managed this a few days before being admitted to hospital for the last time.

The last week of Meera's life was spent in agony as she hovered between life and death, her spirit unable to let go. It was then that her friends realized that the disappointment of not having been able to send her completed manuscript to the publishers was holding her back. On the morning of 26 February 2015 (which happened to be the death anniversary of Anandibai Joshee), they hastened to her side as she lay on her hospital bed and assured her that the manuscript would be sent to Routledge, her publisher. It was only then that she was at peace and passed away before the day came to a close.

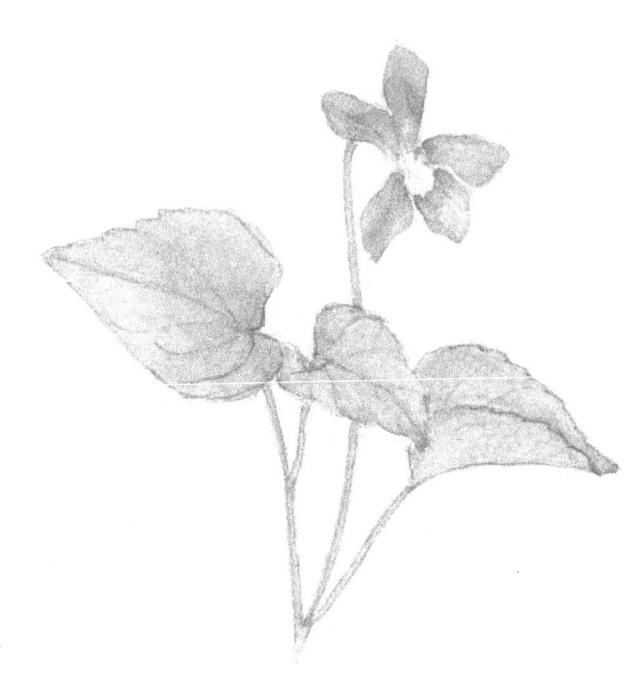

Madhavi Kolhatkar: *Meeratai*

Meeratai, or '*aho* Meeratai': that is how I addressed her from the very beginning. Later (when she complained about a younger person dis-respectfully calling her by name) I came to know that that is how she preferred to be addressed. (It would be unjust not to mention here that after some years she told me to use *e* instead of *aho*.) Now one might say that for a scholar who has travelled the world over, this might seem to be a little conservative; and yes, she was a peculiar combination of modernity and conservativeness, and that might have attracted her to the story of Anandibai. The two of them seem to have shared some similarities. Meeratai was no doubt an independent, self-sufficient woman. On the one hand, she was very free in choosing the attire she wanted to wear, the hairstyle she wanted to have; but on the other, she was very sensitive to what others said (or might say) about her. She could also be very hurt when her father – whom she respected and in many ways adored – was criticised, even though at times he had not been as fatherly as she wanted him to be: D. D. Kosambi was always the scholar. It got more difficult with the passing years, and towards the end she would say that she had decided that her father and grandfather were capable enough of taking care of and protecting themselves.

As it appears from the present biography, Anandibai Joshee did not get much affection from her mother. Even though it was her husband who did not spare any effort to educate her, he had been very chauvinistic at times, sometimes even cruel – Anandibai Joshee mentions this but does not divulge the details. She had a strong sense of social commitment which motivated her to become a doctor to serve Indian women who, because of inhibitions, could not avail of proper diagnosis and accurate treatment. Though very strong and firm and liberated in some respects, Anandibai was very submissive to her husband. She felt guilty to go against him, even when it was a matter of health as, for example, her decision to change from nine-yard to six-yard saris in the snowy winters of New York.

Meeratai was a *gruhini* in the complete sense of the term. She would have *rangoli* made every day at her door. For Gudi Padwa and Diwali, she would get the house cleaned, have the ceremonial lamp lit, and invite people for lavish meals. She followed all the customs a householder is supposed to follow. I remember her bringing a Ganesha coin when she first came to see my grandson. Was it this similarity between her and Anandibai, the combination of being outstanding while still following societal norms, which attracted Meeratai to this project? Perhaps this consonance and the shared values made her try to understand the real Anandibai, and to write this frank and candid biography.

*

I first met Meeratai sometime in the late 1980s. At that time she was a member of the Management Council, Deccan College, Pune. I, a staff-member of the Institute, had some problems regarding my leave, which were to be discussed in the Council meeting. In that connection I had gone to her and explained my case. She listened to it very patiently.

Afterwards we used to meet in the Discussion Group of Law College and also in the National Film Archives of India for movie screenings and walked back together since we lived on the same road. But our really close contact dates from 2007, the time of her father's birth centenary. She had arranged for a series of lectures to be delivered by eminent scholars and would invite me to them. As far as possible I attended them. Then, once she came to our Sunday morning reading session of *Tukaramagatha*. Even though it was not at all successful, our academic discussions continued, even on the phone, in connection with the book she was writing. One day she asked me what the nickname *Ampu* stands for. I couldn't think of anything. Then, after some days, on her own she called me and told me that it is short for *Annapoorna*.

After her book *Crossing Thresholds*[3] was published, she suggested that we work together on women saints. We started reading Bahinabai, but this did not continue for long since she changed her residence and went to Sankul. The discussion group was also not active. In 2011, I was very happy to see her in the nearby grocery shop. Fortunately, at that time she had come back again to her old residence, now the new Vanali Apartments on Bhandarkar Institute Road. Our meetings resumed.

Only then did I speak with her regarding her family. She was very proud of her father and grandfather and would challenge me to name any other personality who was as versatile and as brilliant as her father. While adoring his intelligence and brilliance no doubt, she did have a sense of dissatisfaction and complaint against him as a father. She felt that he expected a lot from her, though her career had always been outstanding. On the other hand, her feelings towards her mother were always of extreme love and affection, bordering on devotion. When my own mother was staying with me, she would demand complete attention and I could not do any academic work when she was awake. I always respected her wish. This, all the more, made me realize what Meeratai had sacrificed for *her* mother. She never accepted any permanent position in Sweden so that she could fly home whenever necessary. It was really a very great sacrifice, for she could not get any retirement benefits. In India she lost the right even to partial pension by just a year. Economically she was sound: She had a very big and beautiful house and enough of a bank balance to live comfortably. But it always pained her that it was the inheritance and not her own earnings. At such times I really felt that she had earned it by sacrificing her career for the sake of her mother, and by the extreme care she took of her mother.

Once, I asked her why she did not marry, to which she replied that she was a perfectionist and wanted to have a very happy marriage and especially very good and happy children. However, as there is only a fifty percent chance of a marriage being successful, she did not want to take the risk and make the life of her children, if she had any, difficult. I wonder if this fear was rooted in her childhood!

The origin of perfectionism was her mother and her grandmother. Her mother would insist that while stitching, all the stitches should be uniform and also while cutting the vegetables, all the pieces should be of equal length. Her mother made her redo her stitching until her work was up to the mark, and Meeratai unquestionably obeyed. As a result, thenceforth whatever Meeratai attempted to do, she did it with complete devotion and perfection.

Being a perfectionist, she was very strict and got irritated very easily when she saw imperfection. But it was not only with others – even with herself she was as strict, so those of us who were close to her did not mind her getting angry. I remember Prof. Ramaswamy hesitating to enter the house with his shoes on even after Meeratai's passing, thinking she would not have liked it. I had to tell him that since we were not able to find a maid at that time, the house was dusty, so he could enter with his footwear on!

Our meetings were mainly centered on academic matters. We had taken up the project of translating the Marathi female saint poets and then began to work separately on the various aspects. She had many plans and ideas. We started with the work of the wife of Chokha, the verse 'avaghaa ranga eka jhaalaa'. Unfortunately, we had to stop after she started having severe headaches.

On her last day in her house, Saturday, 31 January 2015, I was with her from early morning, just sitting and doing my own reading. She was so pleased and said, 'How nice is this feeling that there is somebody in the house who will open the door if the bell rings; and also will come to me if I need anything!'

When I am unwell, I always think of Meeratai. For her being ill signified a state of imperfection, and she would refrain from complaining or sharing her pain and discomfort with others. Not by even a sigh would she let on that she was feeling unwell. When she realised she did not have many years to live, she directed all her energies towards completing her two books: one on Pandita Ramabai and the other on Anandibai Joshee.

On the morning of 26 February 2015, when Meeratai lay in hospital, we, her friends, promised that we would see to it that her books were published. That afternoon, at 2.30, she breathed her last, and by strange coincidence it was the same day on which, 128 years earlier, Dr Anandibai Joshee had passed away.

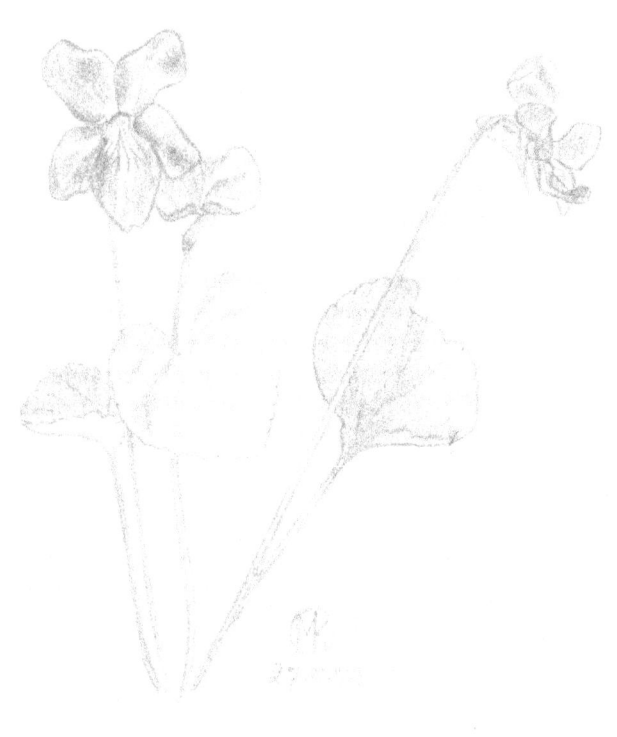

Ram Ramaswamy: *MT*

I became acquainted with Meera Kosambi in 2010 when I started putting together material for a book on her father's mathematics and statistics.[4] Of the three of us this project has brought together, I knew her the least. The compartments that Meeratai had put each of us in – she firmly and quickly insisted on my addressing her thus (so the informal Meera had to become the more respectful Meeratai, which, reduced to MT, was how I addressed her mostly) – were so well separated that I did not meet Aban and Madhavi until much after Meeratai had passed away. Nor had she told me in any detail about them earlier. And she hadn't told me how close she had been to finishing this biography of

Anandibai Joshee when we last spoke, less than a month before she passed away. And of course, she did not divulge the seriousness of her medical condition then.

When I first met her in her Pune apartment, she was most gracious and very willing to share whatever primary material she had of her father's life in mathematics. Most of this is now in the custody of the Nehru Memorial Museum and Library in New Delhi. She was, surprisingly, not very conversant with the extent of the mathematical part of her father's intellectual legacy, and she enthusiastically supported my project. Although much water had flown under that bridge, I think she felt that D. D. Kosambi had not received his fair share of appreciation for all the different areas to which he had contributed.

Since I knew her only in the last five years of her life, my memories of Meeratai are staccato – occasional visits when I was passing through Pune; a brief overlap when she attended a seminar in Hyderabad; some days in Delhi for a book release; and many phone calls to discuss travel, health, and always, books. There was an afternoon when I dropped in unannounced to find her listening to Kishori Amonkar singing from the *Dnyaneshwari*. As the song unfolded, she shared her enjoyment of it, and then gave me the CD to take home. Another afternoon, we met for lunch at one of my favourite restaurants in Pune and had long conversations about her travels to the United States, and my search for the Vidyodaya Pirivena, in Colombo, where her grandfather had learned Pali and spent some years in the 1890s. And another time, she told me that Anandibai's quilt was in the Kelkar museum.

Anandibai figures in a book that I had co-edited, *Lilavati's Daughters*,[5] a collection of biographical and autobiographical essays on or by Indian women scientists. Meeratai was not happy with the portrayal, which she felt was inaccurate and did not appreciate the feminist dimension of Anandibai. I therefore requested her to rewrite the essay for another collection,[6] which she did. But she also told me then that the story of Anandibai would take many more pages and much more effort.

Meeratai had a difficult legacy to bear, and perhaps for that reason, she chose a complex career path. Her choice of specialization, her research topics, and her attention to detail, not to mention the intensity of her work, made her contributions impressive, both in range and in depth. Aban Mukherji mentions her detailed quantitative study of women in Maharashtra, which was originally commissioned by the Census Board. Although she was unable to complete it, this project occupied Meeratai's mind till the end. She knew it was important, and on her last trip to Delhi, she even tried, unsuccessfully, to enlist the support of one of the Ministers of the Government of India for more data.

As both Aban and Madhavi mention, the two incomplete projects that she fretted about until the end were both biographies. That of Pandita Ramabai was finalized the morning that she passed away. The biography of Anandibai Joshee was a project that Meeratai had been planning for quite a while, and although it was not nearly as ready, we felt that it needed to be completed.

In preparing this manuscript, we have been helped greatly in locating references, by Mrs Meenakshi Pawar (from Kashibai Kanitkar's Marathi biography of A. Joshee) and by colleagues at the Knowledge Resource Centre of SNDT Women's University. Meeratai had been the head of the RCWS and was greatly admired for her contributions to Women's Studies at SNDTWU, and we would particularly like to thank the Deputy Librarian, Shri Vilas Jadhav, the Assistant Librarian, Ms Kashmira Dhirawani and Senior Library Assistants, Ms. Mukta Atkekar and Mrs Vandana More, and the Director, Dr. Subhas Chavan. Shri Sudhanva Ranade, Director of the Raja Dinkar Kelkar Museum has been very kind in permitting us to photograph the invaluable quilt embroidered by Anandibai, and which was presented to the Museum by Wrangler Paranjpye. Dr Joanne Murray, Director and Matt Herbison, Archivist, of the Legacy Center: Archives & Special Collections of the College of Medicine, Drexel University have been extremely helpful and generous in granting us permission to reproduce valuable letters and photographs in their collection. Radhika Jaykar Herzberger went through the manuscript and made comments and suggestions.

Beyond a careful reading of the text and some editorial effort, our intervention has been minimal. All of us are very happy to have been associated in this effort to see that Meeratai's last project reached completion.

This, then, is the life of Anandibai Joshee, in Meera Kosambi's telling.

Notes

1 The Shreemati Nathibai Damodar Thackersey Women's University in Mumbai, usually abbreviated as SNDTWU, was established in 1916 as the first women's university in India.

2 Meera Kosambi, *Pandita Ramabai*, London: Routledge India, 2016.

3 Meera Kosambi, *Crossing Thresholds: Feminist Essays in Social History*, Hyderabad: Orient Blackswan, 2011.

4 R. Ramaswamy, Ed., *D. D. Kosambi: Selected Works in Mathematics and Statistics*, New Delhi: Springer India, 2016.

5 R. Godbole and R. Ramaswamy, Eds., *Lilavati's Daughters*, Bangalore: Indian Academy of Sciences, 2008.

6 R. Ramaswamy, R. Godbole and M. Dubey, Eds., *The Girl's Guide to a Life in Science*, Bangalore: Indian Academy of Sciences, and New Delhi: Zubaan, 2012.

INTRODUCTION

A Fragmented Feminism: The Life and Letters of Dr Anandibai Joshee sets out to reveal the real Anandibai, India's first woman doctor, by peeling off, one by one, the layers of myth surrounding her tragically short life. Its aim, states the author, 'is to retrieve whatever we can of her life and times'. And she invites her readers to participate in that quest. Meera Kosambi 'tells her story through the feminist lens, and so captures Anandibai's character in the cultural milieu of her times'.[1]

Kosambi does not hide the fact that her interest in Anandibai had a personal dimension to it, as she happened to be from the same region as her subject and mirrored many of her qualities. Though separated by almost a century, an invisible bond seemed to draw Kosambi to explore and delve into the life of Anandibai Joshee and bring to life the many-faceted personality of this remarkable woman.

The author identified with her subject on many levels. Like Anandibai, she, too, had to struggle to master English, as her schooling was entirely in Marathi. Just as Anandibai had to live up to the expectations of her husband, so too did the author have to live up to her father's exacting standards. The grit and determination Anandibai exhibited in overcoming all obstacles resonated with the author's own life, where every success was wrung out of personal trials and tragedies. Like Anandibai, Kosambi was intrepid and proud of her cultural heritage. She meticulously observed cultural customs yet exhibited a remarkable degree of freedom of thought and action. In this work Kosambi combines vigorous scholarly objectivity with a passionate identification with her subject, enabling the reader to become aware of the many strands woven into the rich fabric of Anandibai's life.

*

When myths are created around the life of a person and biographies are written to perpetuate those myths, truth is likely to take a back seat.

Over the years such retellings tend to perpetuate the lie (based on the author's own prejudices and predilections), and in spite of evidence to the contrary, tend to overshadow the truth.

The patriarchal retellings of Anandibai's story have done a great disservice and injustice to her by portraying her as a passive Galatea to her husband Gopalrao's Pygmalion, thereby robbing her of agency and independent thought. But it has to be said that unlike Pygmalion's creation, Anandibai was 'no passive creature; she played a vital role in her own transformation. In fact it was a flowering rather than a transformation'.[2]

Anandibai Joshee was born at a time when the Social Reform Movement in Western India was in full swing. The spread of Western education in India, through government schools as well as mission schools in the nineteenth century, opened up a whole new universe of ideas which began a train of enquiry and introspection culminating in a forceful reaction against colonial rule.

The first generation of English-educated youth was full of admiration for Western learning, which encouraged a spirit of freedom. The colonial gaze was often overtly racist in its strident criticism of all things Indian, thereby forcing students to reflect on concepts long taken for granted. Many now began to view their culture and traditions with a more critical eye, defending the core values of Indian civilization while daring to voice their opposition to the many reprehensible customs that debased it.

By the middle of the nineteenth century, the Reform movement was at its zenith. Voices were raised and action taken against caste oppression as well as child marriage and enforced widowhood. Liberals like Dadabhai Naoroji, Behramji Malabari, G. G. Agarkar, Justice Ranade, and R. G. Bhandarkar were at the forefront of this battle, demanding education for women as a means of improving their pitiable condition, especially those of the upper castes whose every action was proscribed by notions of ritual purity and pollution. These young men were full of admiration for companionate marriages and wanted their illiterate wives to gain an education so that they could share in their intellectual interests as well as become better homemakers.

The orthodox faction, often anti-British to the core, was vociferous in its demand for political freedom at the cost of social reform. Nationalism was pitted against Westernization, and any criticism of Indian social practices was considered tantamount to a betrayal of the motherland.

The Social Reform Movement was from the start a male-dominated project, and any direct or vocal participation of women as individuals in their own right was frowned upon. Many of the reformers were deeply ambivalent about the outcome of the reforms they themselves advocated, and the concept of gender equality was viewed with suspicion as a threat to patriarchal power. Most of them never managed to internalise this very alien concept of freedom of thought, choice, or action. Such deep rooted insecurity and anxiety led many reformers, such as Anandibai's husband, Gopalrao Joshee, to backtrack from or vacillate between the orthodox and reformist camps, propagating the education of women and widow remarriage one moment and then extolling child marriage.

It is truly remarkable how this male-dominated bastion was breached by such exceptional women as Anandibai Joshee, Pandita Ramabai, Kashibai Kanitkar, and Savitribai Phule. In the case of Anandibai Joshee, though led by her much older husband, Gopalrao, to pursue the path of education, the child bride showed remarkable aptitude in grasping difficult subjects; and her independence of spirit led her to think for herself. An ardent nationalist, Anandibai longed to help her more unfortunate sisters by acquiring a medical education to ameliorate their plight. It was this that led her to the United States to study medicine at the Woman's Medical College of Pennsylvania (WMCP) in 1883. While Gopalrao was publicly fêted for his wife's achievements, he often contemplated abandoning the Indian cause for the glamour of the West, vacillating between remaining in America after his wife's graduation, urging her to practise her vocation there, and returning to India. Anandibai remained firm on this score and threatened to return alone to India.

As a nationalist, Anandibai found her American experience positive, fulfilling, and exhilarating in many ways, but also fraught with tension. Privately acknowledging many of the virtues of the West, she felt compelled to defend her culture; and her pride in her Brahmin lineage made her publicly defend its shortcomings, thus earning the praises of the orthodox faction as well. She was held up as the perfect foil to Pandita Ramabai, whose conversion to Christianity was seen as a betrayal of her motherland.

In America, Anandibai scrupulously followed all the rituals and practices of her caste, abstaining from eating flesh and remaining true to her religion. It was a balancing act which proved to some extent detrimental to her already-failing health and well-being. But it also imbued her with the conviction of the benefits of amalgamating the best of Western medical practices with traditional Ayurvedic ones, and if she had lived longer, she could have become 'the pioneering doctor who combined modern Western and traditional Indian medical systems'. [Chapter 12]

*

Only a handful of women like Anandibai Joshee could rise above such societal pressures to express their individuality, and only a minuscule number succeeded in living life on their own terms. The majority of women were overwhelmed by the restrictions placed on them by their patriarchal society. (Tagore's short story *Exercise Book*, a sensitive portrayal of the plight of a young girl whose desire to learn is completely squashed by society, shows the commonality of suffering experienced by women in different parts of India.) Often, the child wife, having just entered puberty, her body not yet physically ready for childbirth, trying to adjust to the alien atmosphere of her marital home, was torn between her reformer husband's expectations; his admiration for the ideals of womanhood embedded in Western thought, which he tried to thrust upon her; and the grim reality of relentless disapprobation shown by the womenfolk of the household, ready to place hurdle after hurdle in her path to modernise herself to please her husband. Reformers desired their wives to be ideal homemakers. A wife was expected to be cultured and educated enough to be a true companion to her husband. She should be a loving and dutiful wife who would never overstep her station in life and remain grateful to him for educating her without ever being aware of the cruelty exhibited by his own family members towards her.

It is truly amazing how these women managed to hold their own when the odds were so heavily stacked against them.

*

The life of an individual cannot be divorced from the context of her times. But neither can one ignore an individual's unique attributes, qualities and faculties, and the distinctive characteristics that make up the personality – the will or agency that drives her to act independently of social pressures, the courage to deal with or go against social norms and stand up for her ideals.

Born into a Chitpavan Brahmin family, Anandibai Joshee experienced a childhood marred by the harsh treatment meted out to her by her mother, who failed to show her any warmth or affection. To be fair to her mother, such treatment was not uncommon amongst families anxious to stamp out all traces of a free spirit from a girl's psyche, lest she suffer cruelty at the hands of her in-laws.

Anandibai was married off to a man much older than herself who prided himself on being a reformer doing his best to educate his child bride. This stance won him numerous accolades from his contemporaries as well as the undying gratitude of his young wife, in spite of the many indignities she had to suffer at his hands. Many who wrote about Anandibai underplay her own contribution towards acquiring an education. Though still a child, she, too, had the determination and patience to work towards her goal of becoming a doctor, and being a woman, render great service to the majority of Indian women unable or unwilling to go to a male physician.

*

Anandibai's relationship with her husband was complex. We owe the amazingly mature self-analysis of her marriage, though still in her teens, to the distance placed between the couple on account of her going to the United States to study medicine. From the safety of a loving, liberal American home, Anandibai could examine the different facets of her young life and marriage and express her feelings with unexpected lucidity and candour. Without bitterness, Anandibai could point out Gopalrao's often inhuman treatment of her and at the same time express her love and longing for him to be near her. And, surprisingly, these feelings were often expressed in the most ardent terms, indicating her need for his physical presence. Many older women might have been crushed by Gopalrao's harsh treatment, both physical and mental, but Anandibai's equanimity and calm, her ability to think clearly, her nobility of spirit, and maturity far beyond her age helped her retain her sanity.

From the distance of another country, separated by oceans, Anandibai began to perceive her life and her position as an upper-caste Hindu woman of Maharashtra in a clearer light but felt obliged to defend all things Indian in the face of Western criticism. This often put her in an impossible situation and dismayed her numerous American well-wishers who, nevertheless, could understand her dilemma.

Gopalrao's moral vanity; his wavering reformist ideals, keeping one foot in the orthodox camp while professing to be a reformer; his opportunistic behaviour; and his gross ingratitude towards their American benefactors were all additional forms of torture inflicted on his wife. He publicly railed against the Americans and their culture when he joined Anandibai in the United States, but was ready to drop his professed nationalism to settle down in America, a proposal vehemently opposed by his wife.

This leads us to view Gopalrao in a very different light – vain, shallow, publicity hungry, frustrated, and ungrateful. These aspects of his character were ignored or excused by later writers to perpetuate the myth of a caring, fatherly husband, anxious to do his best for his wife. That his treatment of her could have hastened her death has never before been considered by her numerous biographers. In the popular imagination, Gopalrao appears to be an ardent social reformer, and his later slide back into the orthodox camp is conveniently elided.

While it can be argued that Kosambi's feminist leanings are responsible for showing Gopalrao in an unsympathetic light, the discerning reader will not fail to appreciate the extensive use of primary sources and material on which the text rests.

*

Anandibai died of tuberculosis just before her twenty-second birthday. Many blamed her death on the American climate and the hardships she suffered due to her determination to follow her customary lifestyle and diet in spite of her failing health. Her body was, however, already weakened before she had arrived there, most probably because of early marriage and childbirth. Her only child, a son, died soon after birth and left her almost an invalid, but she bore her suffering with great fortitude. Blinding headaches and debilitating fevers were her constant companions.

In America, in fact, she was surrounded by love, care, and understanding, such as she had never experienced as a woman in India. The Carpenter family, though of modest means, showered her with warmth and generously opened their home to her, accepting her as part of their family. Mrs Carpenter, her dear 'Aunt', was more of a mother to her than her own biological parent.

Anandibai felt cocooned and secure in the liberal atmosphere of the land and buoyed by the generosity shown to her. Colleges vied with one another to get her to enrol in their courses. Rachel L. Bodley, Dean of the WMCP, took a personal interest in Anandibai's welfare and looked after her personally when she was too ill to live on her own. It was only because of the warmth and generosity that she received in America that she could survive and complete her medical education.

Her course was very exacting and exhausting, and she had to summon all her inner reserves of strength to soldier on until the end. The strain of mastering English was so great that she temporarily forgot Marathi (thereby inviting the wrath of her husband instead of his sympathy). But she gained in maturity and wisdom, her intellect honed by the sharp intensity of her studies. She could lucidly articulate and convey her thoughts to large audiences. She found that Americans had an open mind and were willing to learn about her country and its culture. They were respectful of her customs and displayed no overt racism in their attitude towards her – a contrast to the many indignities she and her husband had suffered at the hands of their British masters.

As Anandibai grew in intellectual stature, she became more respectfully independent in her thoughts and actions vis-à-vis her husband and was unafraid to make painful decisions. She could publicly defend herself and her nation and was very clear as to what she wanted to do in the future. By the end of her brief life she had outstripped her much older husband both in intellect and in integrity, remaining still the quintessential *pativrata*, or dutiful wife, ever grateful for the path of education her husband had opened up for her.

Anandibai passed away soon after she returned to India, full of hope and determination to serve her suffering sisters. Her untimely death was mourned on two continents and her ashes were sent to America to be placed in the Carpenter family vault.

It is the brief life of this extraordinary woman, Anandibai Joshee, which the author attempts to fathom and present to the world in its richness and complexity.

Aban Mukherji
10 January 2018

Notes

1 Comment made by a discerning reader who wishes to remain anonymous.
2 Ibid.

INTRODUCTION

It was an emotionally charged and in fact, a stunningly close encounter with Anandibai Joshee which I had in the winter of 1995 as I stood before her grave marker. This distinguished and sadly short-lived Indian woman achiever of the nineteenth century (1865–1887), from my own home province of Maharashtra in Western India, was almost palpably present in that moment in the United States – she in a sense a permanent resident straddling two worlds in death as in life, and I a visitor. It was a moment that makes one choke with feeling.

The grave marker stood in the final resting place of Anandibai's American 'aunt', Mrs Carpenter, and her family, with whom she had forged a durable link of affection and an abiding closeness. The little stone was partly shrouded in snow, in the middle of the Poughkeepsie Rural Cemetery in upstate New York, which presented a bleak landscape of white ground and a grey sky laced with bare, leafless black tree branches. The fraught moment captured the intense but criminally wasted dedication that was the sum total of this 'first Brahmin woman' who obtained an education – a medical education – abroad. What died prematurely with her was not just her own dream of providing sorely needed healthcare for her ailing compatriot women, but also Maharashtra's emergent hopes for tremendous strides in gendered social progress and, in a smaller way, in the prevalent and mostly conservative thinking about the propriety of giving education, especially professional education, to women.

What this book seeks to present is Anandibai's life stitched together from various sources, a reconstruction of her personality, and a retrieval of her social milieu. The bare outline of Anandibai's life starts with her customary child marriage, a pregnancy at twelve, a child delivered but lost after only ten days, no subsequent pregnancies, and the sublimation of all her energies into studies at the insistent tutelage of her widower-husband, Gopalrao, who was seventeen years her senior and

1

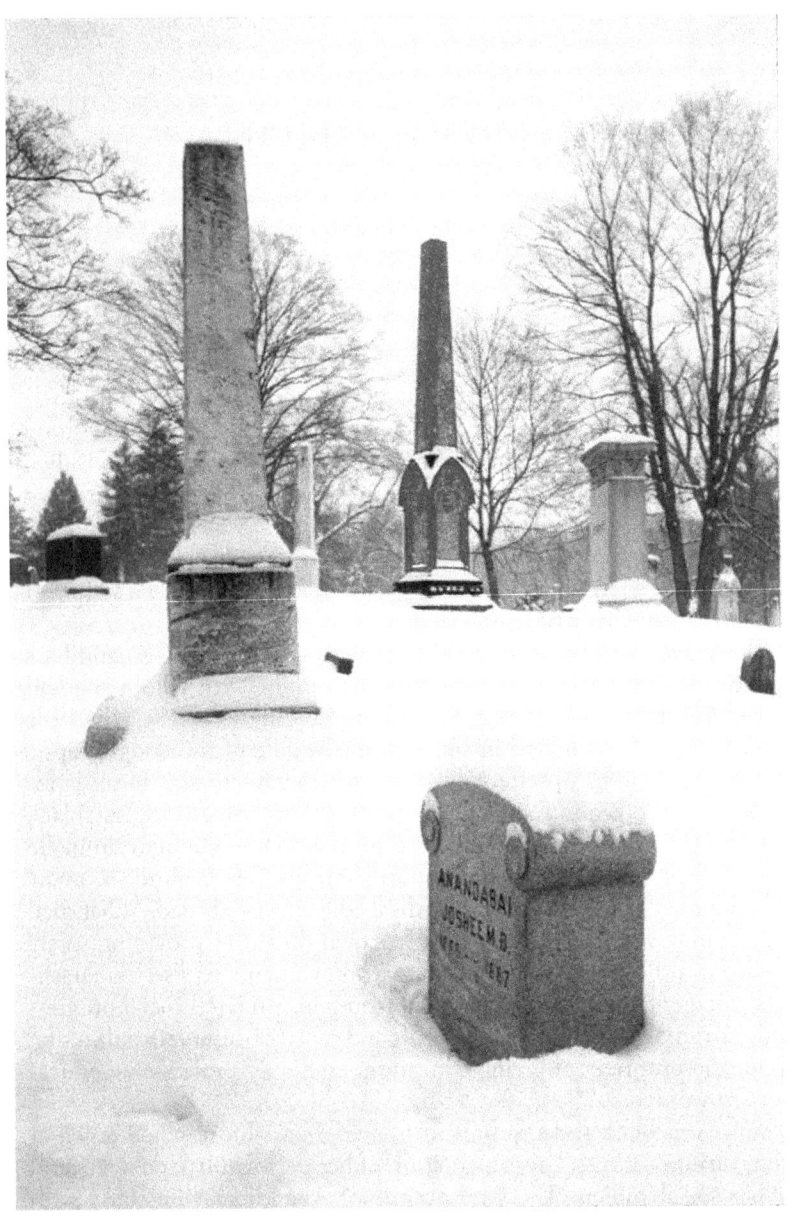

Figure I.1 Anandibai's grave marker (foreground) in the Poughkeepsie Rural Cemetery, New York, winter 1995.

Source: Photograph by the author

filled with vicarious ambitions. Gopalrao Joshee's transferable job as a postmaster in the Bombay Presidency took the couple from Kalyan to Mumbai, Kolhapur, and then Bhuj (now in Gujarat). From Kolhapur, Gopalrao wrote to a missionary, an Indian veteran, then living in Princeton, New Jersey, seeking his help to take Anandibai to the United States for further studies. The missionary did not oblige, but published the correspondence in *The Missionary Review*. Months later, Mrs Carpenter of Roselle, New Jersey, happened to read it. Her generous heart went out to Anandibai and she wrote immediately to offer help. Thus started a regular correspondence, and the friendship ripened into a warm surrogate relationship of 'aunt' and 'niece'. Gopalrao transferred to the Bengal Presidency for certain benefits and it was from there that Anandibai finally left India in April 1883 for Poughkeepsie, New York. With Mrs Carpenter's help she enrolled in the Woman's Medical College of Pennsylvania, completed the four-year course in three years, and started an internship in Boston, Massachusetts. But her chronically poor health had by then been attacked by tuberculosis, incurable at the time. Fortunately, she was offered the post of doctor in the princely state of Kolhapur. She returned in late 1886 along with her husband who had arrived in the United States for her graduation that March. By the time she reached India, she was quite ill. Medical treatment from Western and traditional Indian physicians offered no cure, and she died in February 1887, one month short of her twenty-second birthday. She was cremated at Pune with religious rites. Her ashes, sent by Gopalrao to Mrs Carpenter, are now buried in a cemetery in Poughkeepsie, NY.

This life has been sketched with various fanciful touches by quite a few writers for their own intriguing motives. Her first biography – immediately after her death – came from Caroline Dall (1888), an American feminist author who knew her for three years in America but did not understand her Indian milieu and has therefore misrepresented her in some ways.[1] Dall's hegemonic and even racist position is clear from her comments, such as 'a little brown baby' to describe infant Anandibai, or 'when her yellow face lights up' to describe Anandibai's animation.[2] Dall was motivated partly by her interest in Anandibai, but also by her admiration for Pandita Ramabai, a relative of Anandibai's. One suspects that but for the convention of writing biographies of persons no longer living, she would have written the life of Ramabai. Dall has cast Anandibai in the mould of 'an enlightened Hindoo woman from benighted India' who sought American shores.

This text partly helped the Marathi biography by Kashibai Kanitkar (1889), a budding and reformist author keenly empathetic to Anandibai whom she had never met but whose life ran parallel to hers.[3] In fact,

Kashibai's biography becomes her personal narrative through the insertion of comments which reveal her own experiences – for example, her debt of gratitude to her husband for the gift of education – which she also transposes on to Anandibai in similar words.[4] For feminist reasons Kashibai wanted the biography to be written by a woman, but none was available and she undertook the task herself. This was the first instance of a Marathi biography of a contemporary woman written by a woman. Kashibai portrays her from the position almost of a devotee as an iconic social reformer and nationalist but primarily 'a conformist wife' who by definition elicited acceptance from her contemporaries.

Later, under the garb of 'biographical fiction', the novelist S. J. Joshi painted her in the 1960s as a timid and obedient creation of her visionary, Pygmalion-like husband, who was well ahead of his times, thus totally undercutting her agency in an assertion of patriarchal rewriting of history.[5] This subversion of her achievement has been perpetuated for English readers by the book's free translation, which has often been mistaken for authentic source material.[6] Additionally Anjali Kirtane has written a Marathi biography, but without attempting to interpret Anandibai in any way.[7] I have suggested my own reading of Anandibai as a somewhat conflicted feminist and as a nationalist.[8]

Interestingly, Anandibai's self-narrative traces most of her sadly short life and is available through epistolary dialogues – especially with Gopalrao and with Mrs Carpenter – which can be braided together.[9] They reveal facets of her personality and the gradual evolution or temporary swings in her ideas and perspectives, in all the spontaneity and immediacy as well as all the inconsistencies that letters naturally inhere. These facets show clear contours of her personality. Almost all the letters reproduced here have been pruned to enhance their readability.

Letter-writing was not a part of an Indian's daily routine. Besides, in an age when women's education or even literacy was frowned upon, it was a near impossibility. The enormousness of Anandibai's unique achievement in this regard will come across from Kashibai Kanitkar's description, based on bitter personal experience:

> If a woman picks up a paper, our elders feel offended, as though she has done something very shameful. If she receives a letter from her relatives, all the family feels dishonoured. If a woman's name appears in a newspaper, if her essay is published, if she stammers out a few words at a women's gathering, she is certain to be slapped with the gigantic charge of having tarnished the family's honour![10]

Thus, the cache of Anandibai's letters is a rare treasure. The letters were obviously intended only for the recipient and not for publicity. Anandibai could not have imagined their being published in a book. They remain spontaneous personal documents, not self-consciously crafted and polished. What is impressive about the letters to Mrs Carpenter is Anandibai's sufficient grasp of English, which enables her to describe adequately everyday occurrences, social structure, cultural practices, and shades of feeling – acquired after only a year of formal schooling and five or more years of home-schooling by her husband, possibly supplemented by her own reading. All this yielded a sufficiently large vocabulary. That her English is stilted, at times ungrammatical, at others transparent enough to reveal the original thinking in Marathi, has to be condoned. I have preserved her style intact, with only slight corrections. Inevitably the contents of the letters are of uneven interest, except for her social comment and personal revelations. The description of houses, lifestyles, and events are a response to Mrs Carpenter's vast curiosity and read like short school essays.

In every letter to Mrs Carpenter, the bulk is written in a neutral tone, and there is a consistent valorisation of her in sometimes hyperbolic terms. This relationship is not easy to fathom. Mrs Carpenter was obviously a warm, generous person, sensitive to Anandibai's plight as described in Gopalrao's published letter and the missionary's rebuff. That she was the only one who responded, and the flood of positive responses from other Americans that she expected was not forthcoming, says a great deal about her. Her attitude to Anandibai was maternal and caring – contrasting with Anandibai's own mother's harshness to her. There was also a large element of friendship in it, of two persons trying to make contact across multiple divides. Indian women had few chances to mix with women outside the family orbit, and in Anandibai's case none of these women could have compatibly shared her breadth of interest or intellectual curiosity. Significantly though, Anandibai ended up calling the older woman – old enough to be her mother – her 'aunt', thus establishing a surrogate family relationship which still makes many Indians more comfortable than with a mere 'friend'. There was a supernatural element to this relationship as well, as shown by both women's interest in the occult.

Anandibai's letters to Gopalrao are most significant as a source for her innermost thoughts, and for unravelling their complex husband-wife relationship. In a sense the two personalities were complementary – Gopalrao being impulsive, volatile, violent, and not very balanced; and Anandibai being stoically calm, silently suffering his verbal and physical violence (but bold enough on occasion to confront him with a realistic assessment of his behaviour towards her), clear-sighted, firm, and reso-lute about her duties and about her life's chosen mission. As with most, if not all, Indian women of the day, she was dependent on him as the source of her maintenance and physical and emotional wellbeing. Again, having lived together outside the orbit of an extended family must have led to a closeness and interdependence not necessarily found in other couples. Gopalrao's insistence on educating her and making her think for herself, and his reading books aloud to her must also have led to a broadening of her horizons, a development which she cherished and later built upon. She expresses a deep love for and gratitude to him, alongside a clear awareness of his flaws and her own. Whether these let-ters are written in Marathi and English is unclear; they are reproduced in Marathi (and sometimes read like a clumsy translation) in Kashibai's book. Anandibai herself admitted to him on the eve of their meeting in the United States that she had 'forgotten' Marathi, having had to use only English day and night. In any case, I have translated the letters back into English. Also, her first long letter to Gopalrao about her voy-age, which he had published in the *Theosophist*, is in English, and this presumably was their language of communication.

The social milieu that framed Anandibai figures as an important factor in her story because that is what consumed and destroyed her ambition and her struggle, and led to her quick erasure from public memory and withdrawal of support for women's education soon after her death. A woman who would have opened a new era in Maharashtra and indeed in India died an ideological death as well.

This makes it almost obligatory to retrieve whatever we can of her life and times. This book is a search for 'the real Anandibai Joshee' – a search in which the readers are invited to participate.

Notes

1 Caroline Dall, *The Life of Dr Anandabai [sic] Joshee, A Kinswoman of the Pundita Ramabai*, Boston: Roberts Brothers, 1888.

2 Ibid, pp. 21, 115.

3 Kashibai Kanitkar, *Dr. Anandibai Joshi Yanche Charitra (Marathi Biography)*, 3rd ed., Ed. Anjali Kirtane, Mumbai: Popular Prakashan, 2002/1923.

4 Meera Kosambi, 'Realities and Reflections: Personal Narratives of Two Women from Nineteenth-Century Maharashtra', in *From Myth to Markets: Essays on Gender* edited by Kumkum Sangari and Uma Chakravarti, New Delhi, Manohar Publish-ers and Distributors, 1999, pp. 125–160. The wording to describe gratitude here is the standard Marathi phrase: 'A debt which cannot be repaid if I shod my husband in shoes made of my skin for the next seven lives'; Kanitkar, *Anandibai*, p. 10.

5 S.J. Joshi, *Anandi Gopal*, 2nd ed., Mumbai: Majestic Book Stall, 1970 (1968). Inciden-tally Anandibai was never known by this name, although it has caught people's fancy.

6 S. J. Joshi, *Anandi Gopal*, abridged translation from the Marathi by Asha Damle, Calcutta: Stree, 1992.

7 Anjali Kirtane, *Dr. Anandibai Joshee: Kaal ani Kartritva*, Mumbai: Majestic Prakashan, 1997.

8 Meera Kosambi, Dr. 'Anandibai Joshee: Retrieving a Fragmented Feminist Image', *Economic and Political Weekly*, Vol. XXXI, No. 49 (Dec. 7) 1996, pp. 3189–3197; Meera Kosambi, 'A Prismatic Presence: The International Iconization of Anandibai Joshee', in *Crossing Thresholds*, edited by Meera Kosambi, Ranikhet: Permanent Black, 2007, p. 91.

9 Dall spells Anandibai's name as Americans pronounced it and reproduces Anandibai's letters to Mrs Carpenter; Kashibai reproduces Anandibai's letters to her husband Gopalrao; a Xerox copy of Anandibai's letters to Mrs Carpenter was generously made available to me by Mr William J. Cobb, the latter's great grandson, from the Carpenter Family Archive.

10 Cited in Kosambi, *Crossing Thresholds*, p. 174.

Part I

NEW HORIZONS

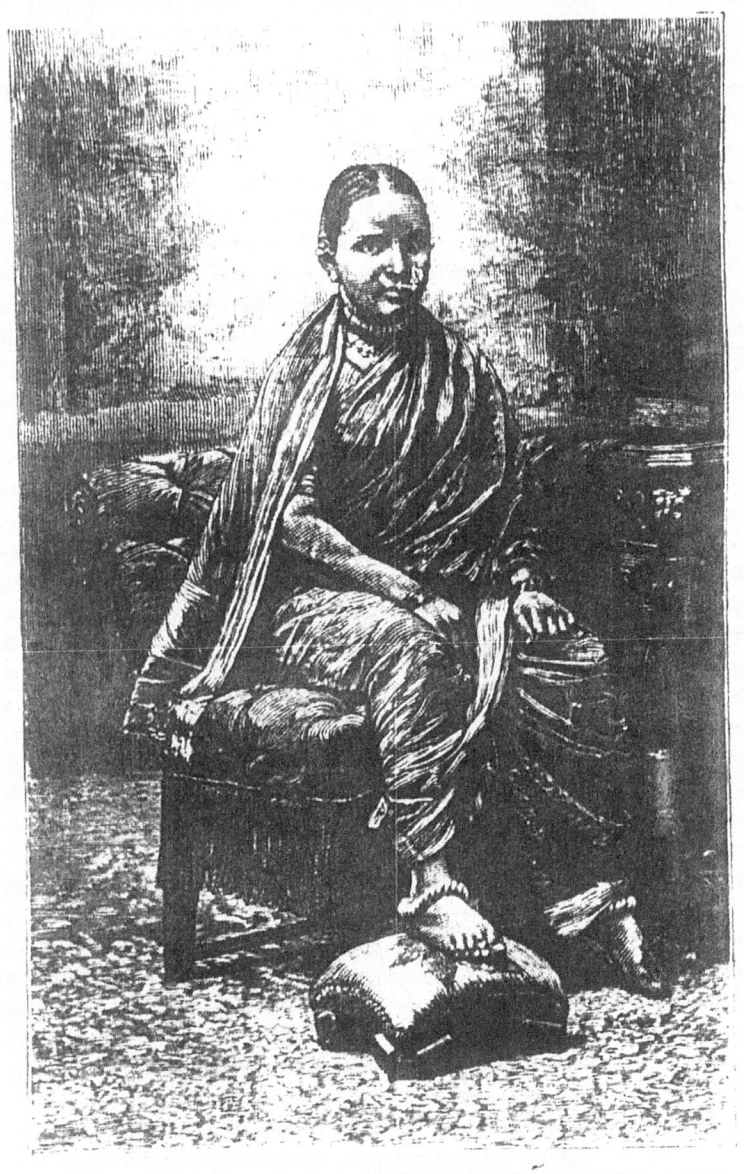

INDIA. MRS. ANANDIBAI JOSHEE, THE BRAHMIN LADY
EN ROUTE TO THIS COUNTRY TO STUDY MEDICINE.
PHOTO. BY WESTFIELD & CO., CALCUTTA.

Figure PI.1 The earliest photo of Anandibai as published in *Frank Leslie's Illustrated Weekly*, New York, 1883

1

EARLY LIFE

The uneasy social transition in mid-nineteenth-century Maharashtra pivoted on Mumbai, the British power centre, rippling out into the rest of the region. Within its purview came the nearby seaport of Kalyan, about forty miles northeast of Mumbai, once bustling with coastal and maritime trade and legendary for its prosperity. But the town's fortunes had dropped steadily with the decline of Maratha power in 1818, and were matched by the family of Ganpatrao Joshi, whose ancestors had formerly been rewarded with a great landed estate by the Peshwa. The once stately family mansion was now reduced to dilapidation. The loss of political patronage contingent upon the transfer of power to the British had impoverished the aristocratic Brahmin family, which still enjoyed a high status as the landed gentry of Kalyan.[1]

Ganpatrao's kinship network encompassed the erstwhile Maratha power centre, Pune itself, through his marriage to Gangabai after the early death of his first wife, who had left behind a son. Gangabai had spent her childhood with her widowed mother at the house of her maternal uncle, a reputed Ayurvedic physician named Balshastri Mate of Pune, and it was to this house that Gangabai went to deliver her daughter Yamuna, later to be renamed Anandibai. This was unusual in that customarily only the first child was delivered at the mother's parental house, whereas Yamuna was the fifth of Gangabai's nine children. Of these only four survived: daughters Kashi, Yamuna, and Sundara, and son Vinayak.[2]

Born on 31 March 1865, Yamuna was the proverbial 'unwanted daughter'. The chubby and attractive baby grew up in a largely conventional social milieu, albeit with somewhat reversed parental roles. Instead of being the usual strict and aloof father, Ganpatrao was generally indulgent, while Gangabai proved to be a harsh mother whose lack of affection was compensated for by Yamuna's maternal grandmother, who was part of the extended family and to whom Yamuna was greatly

11

attached. Under her loving care, which included a nutritious diet unusual for girls, Yamuna grew into a strapping girl who once defeated an older male cousin in a friendly wrestling bout – an achievement which earned her the nickname of *malla*, or 'wrestler'.

Influenced up to a point by progressive ideas about women's education, Ganpatrao enrolled Yamuna in the small school which was run in one section of their large mansion. However, this was probably motivated by a desire to keep her out of mischief, rather than to educate her, as Yamuna was an active and strong-willed child who spent all her time playing games either with the neighbourhood children or by herself. In spite of her half-hearted school attendance, the little girl proved to be bright enough to master reading and writing, much to Ganpatrao's delight. At a time when a man was discouraged by custom from showing his attachment to his children,[3] he was wont to show off her reading skills to his invariably conservative and therefore shocked visitors.

The tensions which circumscribed Yamuna's relationship with her mother did not stem entirely from the unwelcome disciplinarian maternal duties, but were perhaps rooted in Yamuna's characteristic obstinacy and obduracy, or her being yet another unwanted daughter, or some other personal frustration which Gangabai usually vented through physical violence. Her harshness seems to have been disproportionate. On one occasion, when Yamuna had failed to return home from school at the usual time and was discovered playing with a girl next door, having missed school altogether, the distraught Gangabai rushed out and dragged her home, abusing and kicking her all the way. That this was not an exceptional outburst born of acute anxiety was later confirmed by the adult Yamuna's letter in a moment of relived physical and emotional anguish:

> My mother never spoke to me affectionately. When she punished me, she was wont to use not just a small rope or thong, but always stones, sticks, and live charcoal. Fortunately my body does not bear any scars, and her severe beatings did not leave me maimed, crippled, or deformed. By the grace of God, my limbs survived intact! But oh! the agony of those memories! I don't say this as a result of the emotional distancing which comes about with the passage of childhood. Truly she never understood the duties of a mother, nor did I experience the love which a child naturally feels for its mother. This memory hurts me a great deal. A child which harbours fear for its parents cannot possibly feel affection for them, and a child which feels love for its parents does not fear them. Unfortunate indeed is

the child which has missed a happy childhood. I feel perfectly certain that, having understood the problem, I would be able to solve it. If I ever have a child myself, I will teach people by my own example how children should be brought up.[4]

The emotional scar was predictably permanent in an era when a girl's short-lived childhood passed unnoticed into wifehood and when household duties as part of gender socialisation were transformed without a pause into marital responsibilities, although Yamuna seems to have remained a dutiful daughter all her life.

Perhaps as an escape from this unhappy reality, Yamuna was prone from childhood to occult experiences. Once in a dream she saw a remote ancestor whom she had never seen, and who was identified by the much-impressed Ganpatrao, to whom she narrated the dream the next day. He then seemed to have developed a special respect for Yamuna's power to have these visions, which were to continue throughout her life.

Although possessed of a certain charm, Yamuna was no beauty. Her looks were further affected by an attack of smallpox at the age of five, which left her face slightly scarred, her 'wheatish' complexion darkened, and her hearing slightly impaired. Her broad face, with a somewhat flat nose; generous mouth; small deep-set eyes; and large, prominent forehead, was always cheerful and smiling. A short but well-formed figure and long hair improved her appearance. But in the days when a girl's marriage prospects hinged entirely on fair-skinned good looks – especially among Chitpavans, who cherished the distinctive combination of a fair skin and grey-green eyes – or a large dowry, Yamuna's frame, which made her old for her age, posed a decided problem. At nine she had already become a liability for her parents in view of the mandatory pre-pubertal marriage for upper-caste girls on pain of social ostracism. Handicapped by his inability to pay a dowry, Ganpatrao started a long and hard search for a suitable groom under considerable social and psychological pressures which affected Yamuna as well.

It was thus considered a stroke of good fortune when an acquaintance brought news of a prospective bridegroom in the person of Mr Gopal Vinayak Joshee, a widower of about twenty-six and postmaster at the nearby port-town of Thane.[5] A widower was allowed – in fact enjoined – to marry at any age, while a widow was forbidden remarriage; the bride was in all cases pre-pubertal because of society's moral anxiety that her budding sexuality would lead her astray unless it was yoked to marriage. A couple mismatched in age hardly raised eyebrows, and it would be a few decades before child marriage and the age of consent became reform issues.

A chance visit brought Gopalrao to the post office at Kalyan, and some women of the Joshi family went to the building to peep at him through the rear door and approved of him. Gopalrao was then invited to 'view' the girl at the home of a Brahmin family under Ganpatrao's patronage, and indicated his cryptic approval without the customary 'interview', his only condition being that he should be allowed to educate his bride without interference from her family – a condition unhesitatingly accepted by the desperate Ganpatrao. The betrothal took place immediately and an auspicious date was set for a prompt wedding.

Gopalrao then left for his home town of Sangamner ostensibly to fetch his parents, but in reality to dodge the wedding he had not taken seriously. This incidentally was the first of his many eccentricities that gradually unfolded. When he failed to present himself for the ceremony, much to the chagrin of the bride's family, the priest who had acted as the mediator was dispatched to start fresh negotiations, and was able to persuade Gopalrao to finalise and appear at the next auspicious date. The marriage was finally performed on 31 March 1874 (which happened to be Yamuna's ninth birthday) and Miss Yamuna Ganpatrao Joshi became Mrs Anandibai Gopalrao Joshee.[6]

*

Underneath the twenty-six-year-old Gopalrao Joshee's (1848–1912) vacillation lay not just his usual eccentricity and inconsiderateness, but also some real cross-pressures and frustrations, especially his ambition to make a mark on the reform scene by educating women and, if possible, by marrying a widow. Interestingly, his personal narrative can be pieced together from various sources, especially from his later and partly autobiographical journalistic writings which friendly newspapers saw fit to publish, such as the English-language *Mahratta* of Pune.[7]

As a mature adult he sketched his childhood, with its cross-pressures and shortcomings, which obviously went into the making of a volatile and eccentric personality. By then he had come a long way, socially and emotionally, from his orthodox Brahmin upbringing in the small town – in his view the 'village' – of Sangamner, and his obsessive ritualism inspired by his father.

> In my boyhood I was very orthodox and superstitious like the rest of the Hindus. My holy thread was so sacred to me . . . [that if I lost it] I became restless and uneasy as if I had committed a great sin. . . . I began to fast on the 12th of each fortnight as the day of my favourite deity – Shiva. . . . Besides this I used to observe two other fasting days. My mother did not like this, but she could not

help [it], having no chance to interfere. . . . If it were not for my father's devotional life, I would not have been driven to such rigid observances and practices at such an early age.[8]

Gopalrao offers a vivid description of his appearance on these occasions of fasting and worship: the body smeared with ashes; black beads on his head, neck, and wrists; seated on a tiger skin, burning camphor and incense; waving a platter of lights before the Shiva image, with articles of worship and the requisite flowers and leaves scattered around him. This Hindu orthodoxy was inevitably to clash with the gradually encroaching Westernisation. Like countless similarly situated boys, Gopalrao found his vernacular schooling to be a source of deep inferiority when faced with the confidence bred by a privileged English education:

It was my idea that howsoever learned one was in his own vernacular, he was ignorant if he did not know English.[9]

How anxious I was to learn [the] ABC of the English tongue, I cannot tell. My energies were exhausted on the acquisition of this new language. Nothing but this was before me. To bespeak and write [English] was my great ambition. I thought I would be a prodigy if I knew that.[10]

The intensity of the ambition was fuelled by the visit of his old school friend who had gone to Mumbai and learnt English.

He had become a gentleman and I had remained a fool. His expression and style of walk[ing] and stand[ing] were altogether refined. He appeared to me a 'Bada Sab' [a high-status man]. Though I was his schoolmate yet I had not the courage to go before him, because I looked like a villager, a jungly [unrefined] fellow. I was full of remorse and mortification. . . . [and thought of] suicide.[11]

The feeling of worthlessness was aggravated by his father's derogatory comparison of young Gopal with this clever and smartly turned out Mumbai friend. Gopal was stung into a resolve to overcome the numerous and obvious difficulties to acquire an English education. But, like most children, he was afraid of speaking to his father and strategically used the mediation of his mother by threatening dire consequences if he was not sent to Pune to learn English. The father, burdened with the responsibility of maintaining a household of about six, finally yielded to pressure and borrowed money to send Gopal to Pune for a year. With a meagre allowance, Gopal could afford only the Mission School in Ravivar Peth, Pune, attended by about four hundred boys. The enormous pressure to do well proved counter-productive; he became sick and returned home. This boyish lack of perseverance was perhaps natural in view of the acute financial pressures, although impulsive behaviour and an inability to take a firm stand continued to characterise him in adult life.

Meanwhile, his burning desire to learn English remained. He approached a relatively affluent older cousin for support and funding, but the cousin transferred the matter to Gopal's mother-in-law. He had been married at eleven to a girl of five from the Ketkar family of Nashik; now he became 'a caged son-in-law' and was forced to submit to constraints and discipline for the first time.[12]

Earlier, Gopal's orthodox father had been progressive enough to include his daughter – Gopal's older sister Mathura – in the Marathi lessons he gave the boy at home. The intelligent girl outshone Gopal in studies, and this had angered him once enough to tear up her books in a fit of envy.[13] However, the experience also revealed to him how bright and receptive girls could be, and he later tried to teach his unenthusiastic wife at home, finally prevailing upon his brother-in-law Bapusaheb Ketkar, alias N.G. to continue until she was able to drop him routine letters when he was away. She remained a conventional woman and died early, leaving behind a son who was probably raised by the Ketkars. Gopalrao's close friendship with Bapusaheb Ketkar long survived his wife's death.

Armed with an English education from Nashik, Gopalrao first got a job as a subordinate of the Inspector of Post Offices, was later appointed as a clerk at the General Post Office at Mumbai, and subsequently was given independent charge of the post office at Thane. During the mental depression following his wife's death, he decided not to remarry, but rather to exert himself in the cause of women's education. Later he began to toy with the idea of marrying a widow and educating her, thus achieving a dual reform as a lesson to the 'preaching reformers' of the day. With this intention he had initiated a correspondence with Vishnushastri Pandit, the pioneer of the widow remarriage movement in Maharashtra, who was based at Pune.

Gopalrao's consent to marriage with Yamuna was casual, more a matter of respect for the elderly Ganpatrao, and he tried to escape immediately by prolonging his stay at Sangamner until after the wedding date. Here he played a dual game: He also wanted to please his father by showing his willingness to remarry without actually intending to do so. When it seemed safe enough, he visited Ketkar at Nashik, where the Brahmin matchmaker of Kalyan caught up with him. It was Ketkar who dispatched Gopalrao with some of his relatives to Kalyan to consecrate the wedding at the next suitable date.

*

At the time of Gopalrao's marriage to Yamuna, his domestic situation was quite unusual in that he lived by himself because of his transferable job in the postal department. Nor did he attempt to build an extended household as others in a similar situation invariably did.[14] His inability to get along with people had probably closed this option. After marriage he moved into the Joshi's mansion at Kalyan, from which he commuted to Thane, becoming a resident son-in-law once again, though willingly this time. During the eight months this arrangement lasted, Gopalrao treated his parents-in-law with deference, to the extent of handing over his monthly pay packet to Ganpatrao.

But the new son-in-law's presence in the house had its own hazards. The older women of the family, ever preoccupied with the rites of passage which afforded them the only excitement in their constricted lives, started to pressurise Anandi into joining her husband in his bedroom at night.[15] Ordinarily, the prepubertal bride would be naturally protected from such an eventuality because she remained with her parents until the onset of puberty and was then sent to her marital home in the (mistaken but deep-rooted) belief that puberty was Nature's signal to start married life. It is significant that during the Age of Consent controversy – which started 15 years after Anandi's marriage – the possibility of prepubertal consummation of marriage was ruled out by both reformists and anti-reformists.[16] The anti-reformers further maintained that instead of legal measures to raise the minimum age of cohabitation for girls, the matter should be handled privately through appropriate domestic arrangements. They also claimed that girl brides were roughly used not by boy husbands, but by older remarried widowers. Anandi's case bore out the truth of this even while revealing the chinks in the domestic arrangements.

After entering Gopalrao's room under duress, Anandi would find some pretext to leave again soon enough; he would attempt to coax her to stay, but without using force. Soon the womenfolk – including Anandi's affectionate grandmother – began to complain that if he failed to exert his authority now, she would henpeck him in no time. One night, when Anandi insisted on leaving the room, Gopalrao retaliated by beating her black and blue with a piece of wood lying in a corner. The next morning her back was so swollen that her blouse had to be torn off before she could have her bath. Anandibai was to later remind him succinctly of the incident; Gopalrao himself admitted to being haunted all his life by shame and guilt for the incident. But his verbal and physical violence against Anandi continued; she confronted him ten years later with some of these incidents:

> It is very difficult to decide whether your treatment of me was good or bad. If you ask me, I would answer that it was both. It seems to have been right in view of its ultimate goal; but in all fairness, one is compelled to admit that it was wrong, considering its possible effects on a child's mind. Hitting me with broken pieces of wood at the tender age of 10, flinging chairs and books at me and threatening to leave me when I was 12, and inflicting other strange punishments on me when I was 14 – all these were too severe for the age, body, and mind, at each respective stage.[17]

Such 'domestic' violence – usually unprovoked – was part of a woman's life and could lead to her death in extreme cases.[18]

*

Stuck in the rut of a routine job and lacking the capacity to achieve anything spectacular, Gopalrao found that educating his wife was the only way to prove his reformist credentials. He had made it a precondition for marrying Yamuna that he would educate her. Ganpatrao Joshi, having agreed to it at the time, tried unsuccessfully to resist the actual attempt later. Through a friend, Ganpatrao tried later to warn him of the ill effects of such an enterprise, reiterating the common prejudice that a literate woman was capable of dubious behaviour, such as writing letters to an outsider and even eloping with him. The moral anxiety caused by the idea of a woman evading the strict surveillance she was subjected to by the family was tremendous. Gopalrao replied with his characteristic unpredictability that such an eventuality would relieve him of the lifelong burden of having to support a wife. No more arguments were heard on the score, though indirect attempts to frustrate Gopalrao's plans persisted.

After about eight months of this life, Gopalrao decided to be independent and transferred to the seaside town of Alibag, south of Mumbai, where Anandi, accompanied by her grandmother as an escort and household help, joined him. The Pygmalion-like process of sculpting her personality started in real earnest now, although how far it succeeded, given her own strong views, is unclear. Although spared the constricted atmosphere of an extended marital household, Anandi was under a relatively strict educational regimen – occasionally combined with coaxing and cajoling – and was taught to give up her fondness for bright clothes and ornaments for a simpler appearance favoured by Gopalrao.

It was at Alibag that Anandi came of age a couple of years after her marriage, in about 1876. The event, arguably the most important rite of passage for girls according to the prevailing norms, was celebrated with due ceremony, at which she was decked with ornaments and seated under an ornate canopy. Among Brahmins, marriage was customarily consummated with the *garbhadhan*, or 'impregnation', ceremony within sixteen days of the event, as stipulated by the shastras. Gopalrao had possibly already exercised his conjugal rights, notwithstanding his supposedly progressive and reformist ideas.

Soon Anandibai was pregnant and went to her parental home in Kalyan for the delivery. There, the child mother – about twelve herself – bore her first and only child, a son who died after ten days. The incident was to leave an emotional scar – perhaps aggravated because the infant was a prized son in a society built on son preference. Years later she is reported to have said: 'A child's death does not harm its father, but its mother does not want it to die'.[19] Her conviction that proper medical care would have saved the infant may have been the seed which later germinated into her decision to study medicine.

Early pregnancies were not unusual at the time when immediate post-pubertal consummation of marriage was mandated by custom. Its harmful effects, including permanent physical damage and future barrenness in the mother, were intensively debated during the Age of Consent controversy. However, the connection between Anandibai's early motherhood and her inability to have more children does not seem to have been made. She remained fond of children all her life and obviously expected to have some of her own.

*

Shortly after the loss of her infant, Anandibai began to devote all her free time to studies, at Gopalrao's insistence and under his tutelage. But his behaviour was not always supportive or even considerate, and his temper was uncertain. There were instances of deliberate unkindness and violence which Anandibai was later to recapture vividly, albeit without rancour, in a letter written from America.[20]

> It is not at all my intention to distress your dear heart or cause a rift in our love by raking up old memories. It is very difficult to decide whether your treatment of me was good or

bad. . . . In childhood the mind is immature and the body undeveloped. And you know how I acted on these occasions. If I had left you at that immature age, as you kept on suggesting, what would have happened? (And any number of girls have left their homes because of harassment from mothers-in-law and husbands.) I did not do so because I was afraid that my ill-considered behaviour would tarnish my father's honour. . . . And I requested you not to spare me, but to kill me. In our society, for centuries there has been no legal barrier between husbands and wives; and if it exists, it works against women! Such being the case, I had no recourse but to allow you to hit me with chairs and bear it with equanimity. A Hindu woman has no right to utter a word or to advise her husband. On the contrary she has a right to allow her husband to do what he wishes and to keep quiet. Every Hindu husband can, with advantage, learn patience from his wife. (I do understand that without you I would never have become what I am now, and I am eternally grateful to you; but you cannot deny that I was always calm.) I was born to endure all that. But I am quite content now.[21]

This, the only available intimate account of Anandibai's personal life, shows the seamless verbal and physical violence unleashed first by her mother and then by her husband. If her internalisation of patriarchal norms, requiring a woman's submission to her husband, was strong, so was her realisation that marriage foreclosed a woman's options; her father's doors were closed to her for permanent shelter. Moreover, her protest would dishonour her parental family. Her despair, as that of her innumerable contemporaries, had no outlet except a death-wish. How much, if any, of Gopalrao's violence was intended as discipline for her own good remains uncertain, although Anandibai herself gives him the benefit of the doubt.

In addition to women's education, Gopalrao had other reformist ideas, such as the new expectation of a companionate marriage which educated men were beginning to espouse. In picturesque Alibag he would take Anandibai for evening walks. This was scandalous behaviour indeed at a time when husbands and wives did not talk to each other or even look at each other in the presence of others, either at home or outside. Kashibai Kanitkar records that in the 1880s, when her husband was transferred to the small town of Dahanu (near Maharashtra's current border with Gujarat), the couple and their two children set out in the direction of the sea on the very first evening. The spectacle inadvertently caused complete disruption of a wedding feast when all the hundred-odd guests rushed out to watch and gape at them. The sensational character of these family walks lasted for almost six months, during which shopkeepers would routinely leave their customers and hasten outside to watch their progression.[22]

Tired of this small-town milieu, Gopalrao sought another transfer – this time to Kolhapur, where he also hoped to give Anandibai proper schooling. While travelling to Kolhapur the couple broke journey at Satara and stayed with the postmaster there. Gopalrao met some friends there and went off with them without informing his hosts and returned the following day, unmindful that 13-year-old Anandibai, alone in a strange house (her grandmother having planned to arrive later), was sick with worry.

*

Kolhapur, the largest of the many princely states ensconced within the Deccan Division of the British territory of the Bombay Presidency, had the sizable Kolhapur City as its power centre.[23] Like other princely states, it was controlled indirectly by the British government through a British Political Agent, and the city of Kolhapur had its own British areas in the form of a military cantonment and civil station, the latter housing the city's European community and also the post office where Gopalrao was to work.

Gopalrao's sights were set on the Government Female School headed by the famed Miss Micey, who had arrived from Britain as a teacher for some English children, and stayed on after that family's return home to teach in the school. Although the school was situated far from the post office where the Joshees lived, he enrolled Anandibai there, and later succeeded in persuading Miss Micey, who lived in the same neighbour-hood, to take Anandibai along every day in her own carriage. However, the state officers at the Kolhapur frowned upon the arrangement, per-haps out of envy, and prejudiced Miss Micey to start treating Anandibai quite shabbily. This put a temporary halt to her formal schooling. Gopalrao continued to teach her at home whenever he found time, and prevailed upon the missionary ladies whom he had assiduously culti-vated to teach her English.

Anandibai's rapid educational progress increasingly riveted Gopalrao's ambitions on her to the extent of using her educational needs to also further his own career. He took pains to cultivate the Reverend J. M. Goheen of the American Presbyterian Mission at Kolhapur, often engaging in theological discussions with him, and mooted the radical plan of taking Anandibai to the United States, where he would work and send her to school. Rev. Goheen viewed the plan as a means to serve his own agenda of evangelisation and encouraged Gopalrao to write to the Reverend R. G. Wilder of Princeton, New Jersey. In this exploratory letter of 4 September 1878, Gopalrao presented his reformist credentials ('nothing is so important as female education for our elevation, morally and spiritually') and the extent of the social opposition he faced ('customs and manners and caste prejudices have been a strong barrier to my views being prosecuted'). He ended with an appeal for help in finding him suitable employment to enable him, 'if it please God . . . to take my wife to America for her being thoroughly educated'.[24]

The communication was forwarded to Dr Wilder by Mr Goheen, who had immediately conceived of a grand design in which the Brahmin couple, trained in America, would be key propagators of Christianity in India. In his own covering letter he expressed the secret hope that if Gopalrao 'were to go to our country, he might there be led to renounce all and follow Christ, and I know if such should be the case, there are many persons who would be willing to educate both him and his wife, and send them back to labour among their own people'.[25] The missionary agenda of evangelisation through education was openly acknowledged at this time in India. The Anglo-Marathi Christian weekly *Dnyanodaya* (8 April, 1886) of the American Marathi Mission candidly admitted that '[t]he work of the American Mission falls into two departments, the directly Evangelistic, and the Educational, a difference which is more in name than in reality for the end is but one'. Moreover, Brahmins were much sought after as potential converts, especially since a majority of Christian converts at the time were the lowest castes motivated more by a desire to escape caste-based discrimination and by material gain than by intellectual or spiritual conviction. Brahmin converts could therefore effectively spread the message and function as a powerful wedge into the traditional Hindu society.[26]

Perhaps Mr Goheen's enthusiasm was justified by Gopalrao's oral expressions of interest in Christianity, or even his hints at possible conversion as a calculated strategy to attain his goal. Gopalrao's letter was neutral enough in this regard. In any event, Dr Wilder, with thirty years' experience in India, took a far less sanguine view of the matter and plainly prioritised religious conversion in his reply. He strongly advised Gopalrao to stay on in his country and convert: 'Avow your honest convictions and confess Christ as your Saviour and only hope of heaven, right there among your friends and countrymen, and . . . make the most of your grand opportunity to bring all your dear friends into the same blessed faith of the Gospel'.[27]

In attempting to expose Gopalrao's real agenda through his pretended interest in Christianity, the Mission also exposed its own real agenda of pretending to aid progressive Indian ventures. But Gopalrao's only avenue to the United States was closed.

*

Disheartened by the Kolhapur experience and still obsessed by the need for Anandibai's formal schooling, Gopalrao applied for a transfer to Mumbai, the modern, progressive, and cosmopolitan capital of the Bombay Presidency. As the largest city in India at the Census of 1872 – larger than Kolkata, the capital of British India – it was regarded as the home of opportunities. On arrival there in early 1879, he was put in charge of a post office (with the customary dwelling attached) at Girgaum, a predominantly Maharashtrian residential locality by the seaside. He had come armed with a letter of recommendation from Colonel Snyder, the Political Agent at Kolhapur, to Ms Prescott, who ran a school near the General Post Office in the Fort – the British residential area and also the commercial hub of Mumbai, adjoining the harbour. But the distance from Girgaum was too great, and the school did not provide dormitory facilities, so the plan had to be abandoned.

Finally Anandibai was enrolled instead in a nearby school run by the Society for the Propagation of the Gospel, under the charge of the lady superintendent Miss Dobson who subjected the students to a heavy dose of proselytisation. A couple of years later she recounted this experience to her friend Mrs Carpenter in a letter (26 December 1881):

> If I have at all received any schooling, it was for a year only, when we were in Bombay. It was a mission school. . . . I love these Mission ladies for their enthusiasm and energy, but I dislike blindness to the feelings of others. When I was in School, the lady [Miss Dobson] compelled me to read the Bible on pain of expulsion from the school. When she told me to do so, I told her I would not and came home. I informed my husband of the occurrence and expressed my desire not to go to that school again; but he expostulated with me against the rashness. He said that we would not lose anything by reading the Bible, and brought me round to going to the same School again, where I then abided by the School rules.

In Gopalrao's helpless insistence on sending Anandibai back to the same school, history had repeated itself. As early as in 1842, the Brahmins of Mumbai had called a temple meeting to forbid Brahmin children or adults to attend mission schools – only to capitulate soon afterwards in the face of economic necessity.[28] An English education was essential for good employment under the British dispensation, and most schools were run by missionaries or had an overt Christian influence. What is surprising, however, is Gopalrao's shrewd sense of expediency in the face of his own earlier stint at the missionary school at Pune, which had left a lasting and not so positive impact of Christianity. He later critiqued not only the mandatory Bible lessons but also the school routine and ethos in general:

> I would emphatically assert that most of those who went to this school as pupils or teachers generally slighted or trampled under feet [sic] the sacred teachings of their own religions, neglected the regular habit and discarded the purity of sweet home. Some established and joined theistic churches, some espoused hypocrisy, thus defeating the aims and objects of any party; others became infidels and preached the Gospel of inconsistency as their creed and dogma. . . . As soon as one comes to know or look at [the] English alphabet, so soon does he begin to despise religion and to try to break the restraints of society. . . . Neither his father nor his mother give a thought to the future as to whether this sort of training will lead to disastrous results both to themselves as well as to the Nation.[29]

In Gopalrao's own case, this experience seems to have been the beginning of a lifelong love-hate relationship with Christianity and Christian missionaries. But compelling his wife to continue at the school seems to indicate his implicit faith in her mooring in Hinduism.

Anandibai's ordeal was not limited to her frustrated rebellion at school. She had to walk to school every day, wearing the traditional sari, but complementing it with Western-style stockings and shoes as was done by fashionable Hindu girls. The other girls, belonging to rich families and driven to school in carriages, escaped adverse notice. But Girgaum rose up in arms against Anandibai and subjected her to rude stares, vulgar comments, laughter, and jeering, and sometimes even threw small stones at her to express strong censure. The situation was aggravated by Gopalrao's sudden decision to take three months' leave from the office to go on a solitary tour of North India; he sent his grandmother-in-law away, and then started planning for Anandibai. Finally, arrangements were made for her stay as a boarder in the mission school, but an appropriate Brahmin diet was a problem. None of his friends, when approached, agreed to feed her, because a school-going girl was a liability as far as their conventional family members were concerned. Finally, his first wife's brother agreed, but the arrangement was short-lived because he started being harassed by his social circle. About four years later, while describing her personal experience of obstacles to women's schooling, Anandibai described this harassment in Mumbai:

> Once it happened that I was obliged to stay in school for some time, and go twice a day for my meals to the house of a relation.
> Passers-by, whenever they saw me going, gathered round me. Some of them made fun, and were convulsed with laughter. Others, sitting respectably in their verandahs, made ridiculous remarks, and did not feel ashamed to throw pebbles at me. The shop-keepers and vendors spat at me, and made gestures too indecent to describe. I leave it to you to imagine what my condition was at such a time, and how I could gladly have burst through the crowd to make my home nearer![30]

After a month and a half, Anandibai had had enough of the harrowing experience, and left Mumbai to stay with her parents in Kalyan.

But generally Anandibai did very well at school, and the compulsion to speak English with teachers and classmates helped improve her command of the language. She concentrated solely on her studies, although her grandmother tried to teach her housework. The impression among Gopalrao's relatives who occasionally visited the couple was that Anandibai was conceited. Within the family the reaction was far harsher. Gopalrao's father, on one of his rare visits to his son, was outraged at Anandibai's elaborate schooling. After trying unsuccessfully to dissuade his son from this obstinate folly, the old gentleman vowed never to see his face again – a promise fulfilled by death soon thereafter.

The Joshees continued their daily routine, balancing unconventional ambitions with outward deference to convention as far as possible. Whether Anandibai's continued childlessness, after the loss of her first-born, aroused social censure is not known. Freed from the demands of childcare and ceaseless housework, which tied down her contemporaries within their extended families, she was able and gradually very willing to devote her time and energy to her studies.

Also on the positive side were Anandibai's exposure to new ideas, her ability to think for herself and take a critical look at the society around her (inevitably inculcated by missionary schools and reinforced by Gopalrao's own interest in social reform), and the opportunity to travel all over western Maharashtra. On the other hand, Gopalrao's general behaviour remained inconsiderate and eccentric, as well as violent, as already indicated through Anandibai's own words. But while accepting this violence with resignation and equanimity as an inescapable part of a woman's life, she seems to have genuinely appreciated Gopalrao's occasional respect for her selfhood and attempts to develop her personality. However, the price was heavy in another way. At a time when upper-caste women were protected from contact with the outside world, Anandibai had to fend for herself in many ways. During her frequent visits to her parents in Kalyan, she was made to go to the railway station escorted only by a servant; once there she had to buy a ticket and board the train by herself. Thrown back upon her own resources, Anandibai seems to have become far more self-reliant at the age of fourteen than her much older contemporaries.

Gopalrao continued to feel restless and dissatisfied with the frequent visits of Anandibai's relatives from Kalyan as well as with her own visits to her parents. He was also engaged in a perpetual battle with Anandibai's grandmother, who insisted on teaching her housework, while he insisted on her devoting all her time and energy to her studies. About this time the post office at Bhuj developed a vacancy and Gopalrao was transferred there.

*

On 25th February Gopalrao left Mumbai for Bhuj in Kutch in the then–Gujarat Division of the Bombay Presidency. This educationally peripheral and culturally alien town was young Anandibai's first step beyond Maharashtra. Her grandmother did not accompany her this time, and Anandibai was forced to manage the daily cooking as best she could. Gopalrao was indulgent of her failures and content to go occasionally without cooked meals.

In the absence of a proper school, Gopalrao started giving Anandibai regular lessons himself, including elocution practice. Everyday Anandibai and Gopalrao's younger brother, who stayed with them for a while, were given a topic on which they had to speak at length; failure would result in having to go without food. During the year and a half spent at Bhuj, Gopalrao taught Anandibai Sanskrit. She made further progress in English with the help of one Mrs Batty – wife of Colonel Batty – who also taught her sewing and knitting.

The effect of the cultural exile from Maharashtra was depressing. But the Joshees' loneliness was somewhat alleviated by friendship with the Bhagwats, the only other Chitpavan family at Bhuj, who treated Anandibai like a daughter. A small social enclave had been created at Bhuj in the spring of 1880.

Notes

1 Anandibai's life-sketch is based on Kashibai Kanitkar, *Dr Anandibai Joshi Yanche Charitra (Marathi Biography)*, 3rd ed., Ed. Anjali Kirtane, Mumbai: Popular Prakashan, 2002/1923, p. 12, f.n.2. The honorific suffixes 'rao' for men and 'bai' for women are still used in Maharashtra.

2 Kashibai mentions Yamuna's two sisters, while Dall mentions three.

3 N. V. Tilak, cited in Lakshmibai Tilak, *Sampurna Smriti-chitre bhag 1*, Ed. A. D. Tilak, Nashik, 1973, p. 102.

4 Kanitkar, Ibid, p. 16, my translation. Letters or portions of letters are reproduced in a cursive font.

5 'Joshee' is a variant spelling of 'Joshi'.

6 It is still the Maharashtrian custom to change the bride's name during the wedding to signal her complete change of identity. The full name is written with the personal name followed by the father's (in the case of married women, the husband's) first name, and the family name.

7 This was a conservative paper run by the B.G. Tilak group which was politically militant and socially conservative. Gopalrao had ensconced himself into this faction.

8 *Mahratta*, 16 August 1891.

9 Ibid.

10 Ibid.

11 Ibid.

12 Ibid.

13 Kanitkar, p. 22 This and other personal incidents were narrated to Kashibai Kanitkar by Gopalrao himself and obviously present his uncorroborated version.

14 For example, D. K. Karve and his first wife shared a small apartment with a friend and his family in Mumbai, alongside the young boys among their relatives who wanted a good education not available in the rural Konkan of their origin. D. K. Karve, *Atma-vritta*, 3rd ed., Hingane: Anath-balikashram, 1958 (1928), p. 83. Similarly, Parvatibai Athavale (sister of Godubai who was to be Karve's second wife in a reformist case of widow remarriage in 1893) and her husband shared a house with friends in Goa. Parvatibai Athavale, *Majhi Kahani*, Hingne: Rajhans Prakashan, 2013 (1928), p. 6.

15 Kashibai narrates the incident with great reluctance, with the sole intention of exposing a social evil. Kanitkar, p. 27.

16 The Age of Consent Bill, introduced in the Legislative Council in January 1891 and passed into an act two months later, was the Bombay Presidency's initiative. It stipulated that the earlier age of consent for girls which was 10 years, was now raised to 12 years, both within and outside marriage. Cohabitation with a girl below this age would constitute the crime of rape. For the various aspects of the controversy, see Meera Kosambi, 'Child Brides and Child Mothers: The Age of Consent Bill (1891) Controversy', in *Crossing Thresholds*, edited by Meera Kosambi, Ranikhet: Permanent Black, 2007, pp. 274–310.

17 Kanitkar, p. 188, my translation.

18 See Kosambi, *Crossing Thresholds*, pp. 135–37.

19 Dall, p. 32.

20 Part of the letter has been reproduced above.

21 Kanitkar, pp. 188–89, my translation.

22 Vaidya, Sarojini, 1975, *Shrimati Kashibai Kanitkar: Atmacharitra ani charitra (1861–1948) (The Autobiography and Biography of Mrs Kashibai Kanitkar)* 2nd edn. Mumbai: Popular Prakashan, 1991 (1st published 1980) p. 148.

23 Kolhapur was the seat of one branch of Chhatrapati Shivaji's descendants; the other, Satara, was liquidated in 1848. In the late nineteenth and early twentieth centuries, the much admired Shahu Maharaj was Kolhapur's enlightened and reformist ruler.

24 Reproduced in *The Missionary Review*, 1879, p. 47.

25 Ibid, p. 48.

26 Winslow, J. C., *Narayan Vaman Tilak*: The Christian Poet of Maharashtra, Calcutta: Association Press, 1923, p. 52; Hewat, Elizabeth G. K., *Christ and Western India: A Study of the Growth of the Indian Church in Bombay City from 1813*, 2nd edn. Bombay: Wilson College, 1953, pp. 170, 175.

27 The Missionary Review, 1879, pp. 49–50.

28 Hewat, Elizabeth G. K., *Christ and Western India: A Study of the Growth of the Indian Church in Bombay City from 1813*, 2nd edn. Bombay: Wilson College, 1953, p. 124.

29 *Mahratta*, 16 August 1891.

30 Dall, p. 86.

2

THE AMERICAN CONNECTION

Across the globe in the United States of America, Anandibai had touched a responsive chord, all unknown to herself. One spring morning in 1880, Mrs Theodocia Carpenter of Roselle, New Jersey, sat leafing through a stack of magazines in her dentist's waiting room in the nearby town of Elizabeth, and came across *The Missionary Review* of Princeton. Reading the unusual and absorbing correspondence between Gopal Joshee of Kolhapur, India, who was optimistic about bringing his fourteen-year-old wife to the United States for higher studies, and Dr R. G. Wilder who dashed his hopes, her heart went out to the young aspirant.

Theodocia Eighmie Carpenter (1842–1920) was an educated woman, daughter of Mr Jeremiah Eighmie of Poughkeepsie, New York, and wife of Mr Benjamin F. Carpenter (1842–??), a businessman and an inventor with a technological bent of mind.[1] The couple had two surviving daughters – nine-year-old Eighmie (born 1871), who was christened with Mrs Carpenter's maiden family name, and Helena (born 1874?). Their other children had died earlier: Eldest daughter Viola (born May 1866) and second daughter Sierena (born August 1868) had both died in 1872, perhaps in an epidemic. The fifth daughter, Rosalyn (born 1878), had died in infancy, and son Otis (born 1877) had died at the age of one.[2]

Possibly viewing Anandibai in the light of a daughter born only a year before her own Viola, sadly denied the benefit of an education which she herself took so easily for granted. Mrs Carpenter decided to write immediately to her with an offer of help. But doubt set in soon enough – surely the girl had already received other letters in response to her husband's touching appeal. Surely it would be difficult to find common ground with an unknown girl from an alien country and culture. Mrs Carpenter later recalled her initial reaction: It had surprised her that the 'so-called heathen Gopal should be able to write such beautiful

29

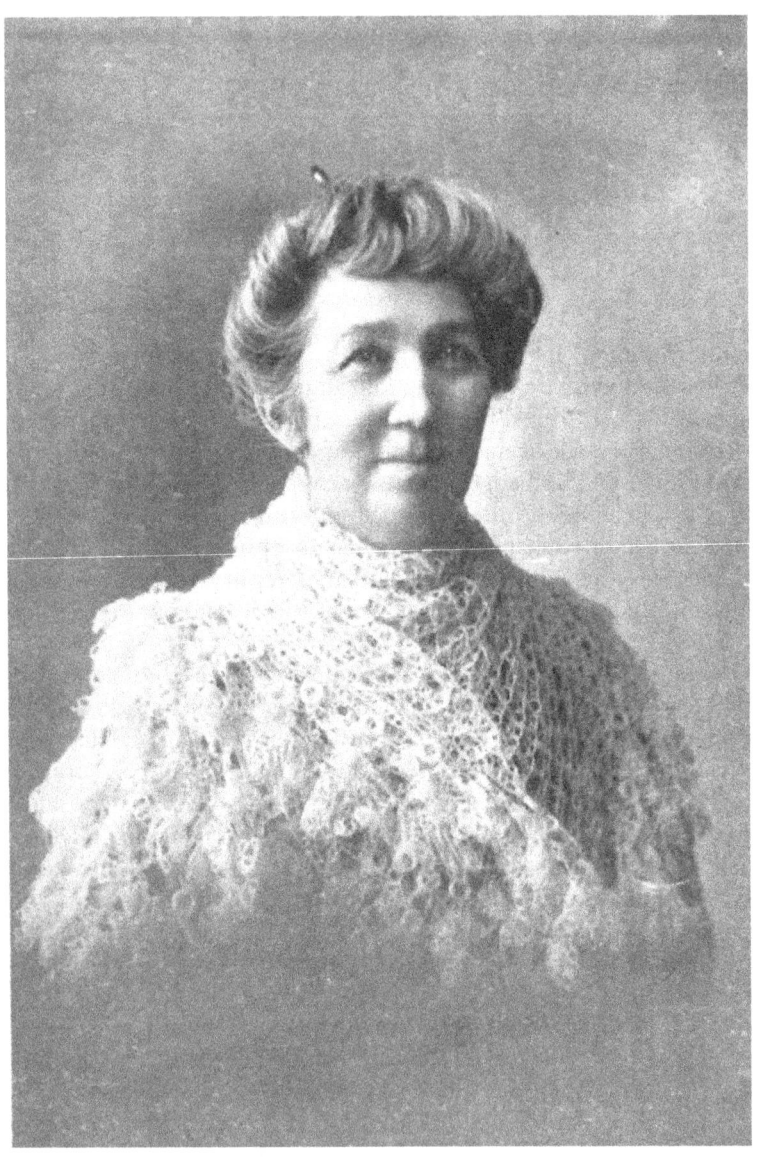

Figure 2.1 Mrs Theodocia Carpenter
Source: Photo courtesy of William J. Cobb

letters, and that his wife should be hindered in an enterprise so laudable for her young age!' The unexpectedly discouraging response from 'an elderly, respected, and eminent person like the Reverend Wilder' and his unconvincing reasoning led her to 'intuitively' imagine their disappointment. Her first impulse was to write to the 'young Hindu woman' and she committed to memory Gopalrao's name and address, planning to write to her. Fortunately, she had not noticed the date on the letter, or she would have given up her plan, considering the lapse of time. She could not even find Kolhapur on the map and wondered whether her letter would even reach. But the half-formed plan lingered on in her mind for a day too busy with other work. Yet the very next day she overcame her hesitation and felt compelled to write the planned letter because little Eighmie woke up in the morning and told her of her dream that her mother was writing to someone in 'Hindustan' (not 'India' as Mrs Carpenter thought of the country). The coincidence was all the greater, for Mrs Carpenter had not shared with the family the letters she had read, and Eighmie had not even seen a map of Asia. Detecting 'a deeper meaning' in this, she sat down at once to write.[3]

Elsewhere, Mrs Carpenter detected divine guidance behind the events. During the same spring, a chance meeting and conversation with a missionary who had just returned from a foreign country, she was inspired by the thought of doing some work in the 'Orient' but without leaving home. The prayer remained unexpressed, but within a few days she came across *The Missionary Review*, followed by Eighmie's remark. 'A letter bearing words of sympathy and encouragement was sent out by the next mail to the little Hindu woman who was living isolated from educational advantages, except such as came through her husband who had little time to give her'.[4]

Thus, Fate, in whose power both parties to the correspondence shared a staunch belief took a firm hand in the matter. On 7 March 1880, Mrs B. F. Carpenter penned her very first letter to Mrs G. V. Joshee of Kolhapur:[5]

Dear Sister,
    I do indeed think of you as a sister, which is why I have addressed you thus.
    We are all children of the same God, and should therefore be ever ready to offer whatever help or encouragement we can to anyone born in a country less favourable to mental progress than ours. When I read the heart-rending letter your husband wrote to Mr Wilder, and when I saw the yearning and efforts to obtain an education, and your strong desire to progress further

than your countrywomen and to help them improve themselves, my heart went out to you and I started feeling a great
concern for you. I can't say how much help I will really be able
to give you, but rest assured that I have a strong desire to help,
provided a way can be found.

Your endeavour is most praiseworthy. I pray to God day and
night that you should see the light of Truth with your inner eye
and enlighten this world, and that other people should also see
the Truth and be enlightened by you.

I consider you very fortunate in having a husband whose
heart is ever concerned about your welfare. Together you can
do great good for humanity. Every place should have such honest, good-hearted, and sincere people. It is often so that he
who is favoured by good fortune lacks an appreciation of good
things and also gratitude. As a result, he is subject to the vices
of selfishness and pride. Your people have many good qualities
which we can emulate. It will be beneficial to understand each
other's thoughts and customs; and the gain will be equal and
mutual because what one lacks will be made up by another!

I will keep on sending you newspapers and magazines from
New York. This will provide you some knowledge about our
customs, manners, books, and intellectual tastes. However,
I think you Indians probably know more about us Americans
than we know about you, because the American missionary
societies in your country surely give you a lot of information.
Besides, after the publication of your husband's letter, you
must have received several letters from people here, and all of
them must gladly have offered information about our country.

Please consider my husband and myself to be your true
friends, desirous of serving you in any way we can. We are in
full sympathy with your effort to acquire an education and
your strong desire to help others. Do keep us informed about
your well-being – it will make us happy. Also, please write to
us regularly about your studies. We always remain students
because the path of progress is unending and moves from the
finite towards infinity.

One should try to lead one's life in accordance with the wise
maxim 'Do unto others as you would have them do unto you',
and love one another. Such conduct purifies the heart and
pleases God who is the source of all happiness.

*

The amazing letter found its way from Kolhapur to Bhuj, catching Anandibai unawares. Her life had been circumscribed by the orthodox Hindu culture – even her husband's unconventionality was rooted in and pitted against Brahmin orthodoxy. Her contact with Americans and Europeans had largely – or only – been through Christian missionaries interested in her mainly as a potential instrument for their own ends. Being suddenly confronted by an American woman addressing her as a 'sister' and expressing a genuine personal interest in her education and well-being across the geographical and cultural divide was unprecedented indeed. Besides, personal affection had rarely come Anandibai's way, except through a grandmother who had been powerless to protect her from harm. A harsh mother and an autocratic, volatile husband could hardly have prepared her for such affection as she had already begun to receive from an American stranger. Anandibai had obviously shared her overjoyed reaction with Mrs Carpenter later.

> Anandibai's hopes had about died out as to all the good she had expected to accomplish through study; and, living as she then was, among strangers, on the island of Bhuj, whose language was foreign and customs dissimilar, the letter from America reached her at a time, when bitter homesickness was added to more bitter disappointment – the letter directed to Kolhapur found its way through several changes of address to Bhuj and she was made so happy that she sang and danced for joy all that day.[6]

The 15-year-old Anandibai immediately wrote a grateful reply which was formal and respectful, without being obsequious.[7]

Bhuj, dated 21–4–80

Dear Madam,
    So I address you as you are my well-wisher and far superior in intellect and learning. I am only fit to sit at your feet.
    Your letter dated 7*th* March reached me yesterday. It has filled my heart with unspeakable joy and a still more growing desire to see the country where such gems are born.
    It is long since we left Kolhapoor [sic]. My husband got transferred to Bombay, but we soon found that Bombay would not supply our wants; the school being out of the way and peculiarly instituted so as not to impart practical and useful knowledge. We were not left alone by society. We had

to struggle against many difficulties, especially social ones. It is only two months since the duties of my husband have brought us here. It is a lonely place, far away from Bombay or Calcutta, where no missionaries can be seen. It is in fact an abode of superstition and orthodoxy where women are but . . . [birds in a cage]. You may easily imagine to what degeneracy India has been reduced. It is, however, gratifying that I am not so treated. My husband tries his best to improve and elevate me that I may do the like towards my unfortunate country-sisters [sic].

Anandibai's incipient feminism becomes apparent from the outset, as does her sense of genuine gratitude to her husband, whose eccentric and autocratic behaviour was redeemed by the boon of education conferred upon her.

I am very thankful to you for your good wishes towards me. My gratitude knows no bounds as you so much as assure me of your helping hand. I shall, indeed, be very fortunate if the almighty God will afford me the means to go to and complete my education in America. I am very anxious to study medicine and serve God and man thereby.

I have not given up my studies. I read English and Sanscrit [sic] with my husband and thus keep up fresh memory that in some future day, I may be able to achieve my object.

I shall be very happy if you will occasionally send me a New York paper or Magazine as you please.

I shall always try to write to you as often as possible and thus strengthen the bond of friendship and earnestly hope that you will do the same. I again beg to express thankfulness for the assurance that both you and your husband are our warm friends and desirous of serving me.

My husband joins me in sending regards to self and husband.

Yours most obliged and attached
Anandibai Joshee

Anandibai's letter heralded a voluminous correspondence: common ground was rapidly established and basic information about each other's country, culture, and customs were exchanged in what Mrs Carpenter was later to call 'a delightful correspondence of three years'.[8] The enthusiastic Anandibai soon lost much of her initial stiff formality and reciprocated the feeling of 'sisterhood' in her very next letter.

Bhuj Post Office
5/7/80

My dear sister,

Your favour consisting of 4 packets and one post card reached me on the *2nd* instant. I am so glad and thankful for it. The more I read and think of your favour, the more I feel attached to you as real sisters ought to be, nay it is more than that, as I look upon you as one entrusted with the cares & management of younger ones in the absence of their mother. My case is the same. Though proud and fond of her, I have no hope of India resuming her motherly duty to give her daughters nourishment. It therefore falls upon England or America to take care of us.

This is the first clear indication of the English-educated Indian's expectation of England and America. India's educational lifeline to Britain had already been established; the American connection was still tenuous. Located within an Anglo-American sphere of influence, the upwardly mobile Indian had obviously begun to expect these self-proclaimed models to own and act upon the responsibility of tutoring the less advantaged. Mrs Carpenter, in a private capacity, had indeed begun to fulfil this responsibility abdicated by the male representatives of the American Mission. She now sent useful reading material about America by way of preparing Anandibai for her eventual visit.

From the reading matter to hand, I am very glad to learn that America is not so orthodox in religion as I was led to believe from the missionary labours in India. Mrs Maria King is really an adept in Hindu philosophy. My religion teaches the same thing. Man is an attribute of God & can attain to divine perfection. One Hindu sage has said that man can become God if he takes it in his head to do so.

Among the many ways in which Mrs Carpenter's letters had begun to expand Anandibai's horizons was the early realisation that the dogmatic missionary might not be a true representative of America and that Americans living in their home country were quite different. Mrs King's description of Hinduism was obviously a welcome revelation of the sympathetic interest in Indian culture nurtured by some Americans.

My husband asks me to request you to send us all the books made by Mrs King and a bill detailing their prices. He shall remit the amount on receipt of your letter.

We have not had so warm weather at Bhuj. We had had very pleasant and cool nights in the month of May and June. Monsoon has now fairly begun in India so that we are now free from warm weather.

I propose to write you once a month say about the 15*th* of each month so that the letter will reach you a week before the time you have fixed for writing to me.

If you write to me in my name as you have done, there would be nothing wrong. I have already told you that women in India are shut up and not within reach of correspondence. But thanks to my husband's good wishes he allows me the privilege of direct correspondence with friends and relatives.

I hope that you with your husband are enjoying good health. As I have my photo lately taken at the special request of my friend Miss Dobson [presumably the missionary teacher in Mumbai], I beg your acceptance of one copy herewith sent. I shall feel obliged if you will favour me with your own.

My husband joins me in sending our kind regards to self and your husband.

Yours ever grateful,
Anandibai Joshee.

Anandibai possibly received some help from Gopalrao in writing these letters; her first letter resembles Gopalrao's own letter to Mr Wilder in its formality and general formulation – though it was perhaps the model learnt in school by both. Obviously, Anandibai spent considerable time and energy in composing her letters, making a draft first and copying it out carefully, as seen from the occasional slips where an entire missing line was inserted later. Even assuming Gopalrao's occasional assistance, Anandibai's strong grasp of English, considerable vocabulary, and articulation remain impressive.

Anandibai's excitement at this new friendship was tempered by an awareness of the gap in their cultures and educational levels; but her modesty and open admiration were untinged by a feeling of inferiority, perhaps due to an ingrained Brahmin pride and the perceived questionability of the Western way of life which surfaced occasionally.

Bhuj Post Office
19/7/80

My dear sister,

Since the receipt of your post card I was anxiously waiting for the next mail which unfortunately suffered detention between

Suez and Aden on account of the steamer having run on shore [sic]. The mail at last arrived on Sunday before last [i.e. 11 July] and brought me your kind letter dated 3*rd* June. I was so much gladdened by it that I thought of writing to you by return post but as I had proposed in my previous letter to address you on or about the 15*th* of every month, I deferred doing so until now, though I could not help reading your letter over and over again every day.

I sincerely thank you for the reading matter you sent me and your desire to know all about me and our customs and manners. It gives me no little pleasure to see that you are so much interested in me but literarily you are so far advanced and naturally possess such varied information on all subjects and we Indian women are so far behind in every point that I am afraid I shall not be able to give anything that you have not heard of before, but it is not so with you, I have no adequate idea about America and her people. I have many things to learn from you, and few to give you in return.

Even so, Anandibai gives an account of her family situation with an easy assurance, and also makes wry comments on the low status of Indian women, which places them outside the orbit of written communication and business transactions, and which denies them even the basic comforts of life. Her independent and progressive bent of mind is evident in her flouting of the custom that forbids a wife from uttering her husband's name, as evidenced by her mention of his full name to Mrs Carpenter.

Incidentally the problem of not being able to utter or mention in writing the husband's name was circumvented in a variety of ways by Anandibai's contemporary women who wrote autobiographies. Ramabai Ranade refers to Justice Ranade as *svatah*, or 'Himself'; Parvatibai Athavale used the respectful plural, 'our men'; Lakshmibai Tilak and Anandibai Karve just used the surname. Anandibai Joshee simply wrote 'my husband'.[9]

Explaining that 'Yamunabai' was the name given to her at birth, and 'Anandibai' during the wedding, she mentions that the former was used in her parental home and the latter in her marital home.

As nothing is transacted in the name of ladies who neither write nor receive letters, it is not required of us to take any designation to distinguish a married woman from a single one except that her name is followed by her husband's full name in documents, namely,

Anandibai bhratar (husband) Gopalrao Vinayakrao Joshee. But now we follow the English in such things. However, in religious ceremonies women have this appellation 'Saubhagyawati' (which means ever fortunate) before their names when they are repeated in giving offerings to God, or in receiving blessings from priests or eldest [sic] persons, when we make them bows.

My family consists of husband, two brothers-in-law, mother-in-law, and one brother-in-law's wife. I had a child which died soon after it was born. We have not much to do in the line of sewing as our dress is homely and simple as will be seen from the photo I have already sent you. We have the same dress for all the seasons. We never put on warm clothes as it is considered indecent nor do we wear shoes or boots as we seldom go out of doors. In short, all these luxuries are for men, who feel cold, heat or rain [sic] and not for women who are supposed to be impervious to all these changes of climate. Should we not envy you then?

This comment on the subordinate status of women, which denied them ordinary physical comforts – treated as privileges reserved solely for men – is typical of Anandibai's sarcastic understatement. Equally significant is her fleeting mention of her lost child, almost slurred over among other factual information, as if the wound had not yet healed, although it is easy to imagine Mrs Carpenter responding with instant sympathy to the pain, having lost four children herself (which Anandibai may not have known at the time). Anandibai's genuine fondness for children now found an outlet in the Carpenter children.

Many many thanks for the photos of your children to whom I send my kindest love and kisses. I do not know what things from India will please them most. Cutch is famous for silver work. Do you wish to have some specimen of it?

The correspondence was regular, and each month a long letter full of interesting details was dispatched willingly and faithfully. The next letter was dated 23 August 1880:

My dear sister,
In my last dated 19*th* July I gave you some particulars about me as you wished to know them. Thinking something about [the] manner of life, caste and religion will be interesting to you, I give the following.

The chief food of the Indians consists of rice, milk, and butter, but the poor are contented with the bread of small maize. We generally love spices in our dishes and being water-drinkers we are very fond of sugar. No Hindu, of whatever caste he may be, eats beef, but the Rajputs or those of the soldier caste eat mutton and perhaps also other viands. No one is more restricted as to food than a Brahmin. He absolutely dares to eat nothing which has had life, and if he wishes accurately to observe all the duties prescribed by his caste he does not even dare to eat onions, radishes and several other leguminous plants, or herbs which other castes have the liberty to consume. All his food must be prepared by Brahmins and the water he desired to drink must be drawn by a Brahmin in his own vessel and at such a time when no other person is likewise seeking water at the same well. Besides we have fast days during one half of the year when we venture to take food only of a certain kind. In short, the obligations of Brahmins are so numerous that there are few in our caste able to fulfil them all accurately without exception. All the Banians [Banias] eat nothing which has received life, but are not so much embarrassed for other nourishment as the Brahmins.[10] In general but few Europeans could be found to live so soberly as the Indians, on the other hand, however, we are also rarely subject to maladies, no strong passions are known among us, although we have also much ardour for working whilst Europeans make themselves by eating and drinking too much and out of seasons not only often incapable of working but frequently draw upon themselves maladies and even death.

The Brahmin cultural pride asserts itself here, as does the common upper-caste belief in the moral superiority of its austere ways, such as a pure diet, which made for serenity of temper, over the self-indulgence and lack of control displayed by Europeans. Personal cleanliness was another source of pride.

The Brahmins have prescribed to the Indians a number of rules on food and drink. We sit down with our legs crossed under us, upon carpets or sofas like the Turks and the Arabs, and at dinner we are so far from each other that not even our garments can touch each other. When we eat we make use of neither knives nor spoons, and have plates which we throw out at the door as soon as the repast is finished – I mean to say large [banana] leaves. When sailors of different tribes have a water jug in common, they do not put it to their mouths when they drink but pour the water direct into the mouth without it touching the lips. To us cleanliness is yet more strongly recommended than to the Mahommedans. We not only wash ourselves before as well as after meals and on certain other occasions, but also every morning and evening bathe our whole body.

Your favour of 12*th* July just received. I was longing for it since it became due a week ago on supposing it was posted about the 1*st* of the month. Your letter is replete with valued information. I am indeed very glad to see you are so usefully employed in things we Indians have hardly any idea of. I shall try to send some vegetable and mineral specimens from India if I can.

I, of late, have been ill with something or the other. In higher classes women generally are very weak in India. I ascribe the cause to the custom of early marriage prevailing in all India, but as you complain of the same, I think there [is] some wrong in the marriage system. With kind kisses to [the] dear little children,

I remain
yours affectionately
Anandibai Joshee

Here is the first clear indication of Anandibai's uncertain health and its probable cause being gynaecological in nature. About this time the high rate of morbidity among women was a topic of general comment, and some years later even the *Mahratta* (1 November 1885) was to admit that '[i]t would be no exaggeration to say that our women, at least in the higher and middle classes, generally suffer from some – one or other bodily ailment.' Anandibai's own vacillation as to the causal link between early marriage and poor health was to continue for a long time in the debate with Mrs Carpenter.

*

The exchange of information had progressed to a general description of the social structure. In broad terms Anandibai was able to convey the gist of the caste system, the rules of ritual purity and pollution, and the diet of the different religious and caste communities and its assumed effects on the body and the temperament. Her obvious knack for capturing the essence of Indian customs in a manner easily understood by a foreigner completely ignorant of India was highly appreciated by Mrs Carpenter, as she told her friend Caroline Dall years later:

> Then began for me, a regular course of education in Hindu manners, customs, religious rites, and everything of interest which her ready pen and remarkable mastery of English could set forth, while I in return answered all her queries. Newspapers, magazines, pictures, flowers, and seed were exchanged.[11]

These informative accounts started almost at once, and the next letter (20 September 1880) was like a school essay on the topic of the uses of the coconut occasioned by a mention of Narali Pournima – a full-moon day when the violence of the monsoon is supposed to have abated, so that the 'deity of the ocean' is propitiated and ships set sail. Anandibai described the coconut as a 'peculiarly Aryan fruit', indispensable on all religious occasions, its water having beneficial health effects and its hairy surface, or coir, used for making various articles. The hard round shell, with the kernel and the hairy surface removed, makes hookahs or hubble bubbles; and half a shell can be used as a cup or bowl. When burnt, the shell yields an oil which has curative powers. The kernel forms part of cooked or uncooked food; and when made into oil, it is used for cooking or as hair oil.

*

Anandibai's mid-October letter seems to have been delayed, again due to the recurrent illness which seems to have taken a serious turn, and which was to run like thread through her letters.

Bhuj
1st November 1880

My dear sister,
   I am late this time by 15 days to mail this letter. It is on account of my serious illness, which confined me to bed for nearly 3 weeks. This sickness confirms me in my desire to study medicine. Though my sickness was not of a serious nature, yet I was at one time so much affected that I had passed some days and nights without the least relief until we had recourse to professional medical advice and treatment. As a rule we Indian women suffer from innumerable trifling diseases, unnoticed till they grow serious. The internal diseases to which women are

naturally liable are never known to anybody except the suffer-
ers. It is thought indecent to let them go to the knowledge [sic]
of the other sex, much more [so to be] examined by male doctors. You may therefore imagine the mortality among Indian
women. If I make to exaggeration, fifty per cent die in the prime
of their youth of diseases arising partly through ignorance and
loathsomeness to communicate of the parties concerned [sic],
and partly through carelessness on the part of their guardians
or husbands. It is not a calamity if a father loses a daughter or
two as he is thereby spared much trouble and embarrassment
to which he is exposed by abominable customs and manners.

This is the first sign of Anandibai's intense and personal interest in
a medical education, as a sufferer denied timely relief. But her sickness
only 'confirmed' and reinforced her desire, which had obviously been
revolving in her mind previously, and which she had discussed with
her husband. Here is also an indication of the prevalence of gynaecological complaints. Of the widespread neglect of women's health, and
an oblique reference to the general dispensability of women in Indian
society in another subtle protest against patriarchy.

Earlier Anandibai had sent Mrs Carpenter her photo, possibly the
same one printed almost three years later in *Frank Leslie's Illustrated
Newspaper* of New York, accompanied by an introductory article about
her. The photo showed her decked out in all her finery, heavily bejew-
elled, seated on an ornate chair with one bare foot (wearing a thick
anklet) resting on a low footstool. Mrs Carpenter's reaction had been
one of surprise: that a woman dressed in such a peculiar style of dress,
wearing bracelets, anklets, toe-rings, and a mark of the forehead should
write elegant English! She was also puzzled by 'a blemish on the upper
lip', which Anandibai explained as a nose-ring.[12]

In return Mrs Carpenter sent her a lock of her hair and some flowers; and Anandibai promised to send a lock of her own hair and some
Indian flowers and leaves in her letter of 1 November 1880. She con-
ceded that the profusion of ornaments might 'appear barbarous to the
foreign eye', but was regarded as a sign of beauty – although the dress
and ornaments changed from province to province in India.

Arguably the most internally troped Indian social customs were
child marriage and the treatment of widows, which naturally figured
quite early in this correspondence – in fact in the above-cited letter.
Anandibai's graphic account of the plight of upper-caste widows displays both her sensitivity and talent for evocative description, albeit in
breathlessly long sentences.

Now I come to your question about widows in India. To tell you the truth, I shudder. . . . [to hear] the very word. You may have many difficulties and inconveniences to labour under, but all that put together in one scale will be like a particle before a mountain in another. Such is widowhood in India. It will be a subject for an essay. I will not therefore be able to do justice to it, but I shall give you some particulars. Young widows of six and upwards are not allowed to marry again. This is not all. They are required to undergo mortifications and degradations of all sorts, besides. A young girl when widowed before she attains puberty must only wipe away the red mark on her forehead, which you will notice in my picture. But when she comes of age she is given a peculiar dress to put on; her head is shaved against her will and desire; all the ornaments on her person are removed; and the glass bangles and wreaths of [black] beads [i.e., the mangalsutra] broken; she is in fact deformed [disfigured] and reduced to a state horrible to look at; she is not allowed to move [about] in society, especially when marriage and other ceremonies are performed; her face if first seen in the morning before [that of] anybody else is a bad omen for the day; if a traveller meets a widow on his first setting out, it is ten to one but that he will return home, and sit for a while before he resumes his journey, but at home she is bitterly cursed by her parents-in-law; she is not given enough to eat; she must not eat twice a day; in short, religion enjoins her not to enjoy life. This of the young widows who have not seen much of the world and consequently cannot sufficiently feel the rigidity of this life, but the case is still worse with grown-up widows. Here the husband is about to die, all the friends and relatives gather round his bed. The dearest and nearest raise a cry of mourning, there his wife, not allowed to join the mourning party, sits in a dark corner; there the mischievous Brahmins contemplate to commence their operation of mortifying and deforming her; there the barber sent for comes; there three or four elderly widows sit around her, not, if you think, to console her but [to] break all the wreaths of black beads about her neck and to hold her fast that the barber may pass his cruel razor over her head. This is the first time in her life that the razor has touched her person. From birth till she becomes [a] widow, her hair is never cut or shaved. So we look upon hair cut or fallen as[13] unclean and do not keep [it] by us. It is not customary among us to preserve locks of hair of our mothers or any dear friends or relations, but as you have been pleased to send me a lock of your hair, I shall do so in return as a special case. You will perhaps ask why shaving is not done afterwards. I tell you that all the ornaments, hair and marks are the emblems of married life and must be buried or destroyed as soon as that state ceases to exist. The hair so cut [is] therefore hurried along with the corpse to the burning ground to be destroyed there by fire. Friends and relations form a procession but the widow alone is left behind and cannot step out.[14] You may therefore imagine the pangs of this bereavement.

Mrs Carpenter later recorded appreciatively that the two still exchanged locks of hair. Anandibai's willingness to flout superstition was indeed surprising in view of the universal dread of widowhood in India, which she admitted to sharing. She had obviously witnessed the widow's ordeal in her family or among friends and relatives; so common was widowhood that practically every family had a widow of every age group. The superstitions related to the disfigurement of widows are also described by Anandibai's contemporaries, such as Parvatibai Athavale, who was about twenty and mother of a son at the time, and Anandibai Karve, who was widowed in early childhood but disfigured later.[15]

Anandibai's partly grim letter ended on a cheerful note with an account of the decorative colouring of women's palms with powdered henna leaves which she sent for Eighmie and Helena, along with some Indian newspapers for Mrs Carpenter, and promise to send 'some articles of Cutchi work' which she had specially ordered.

Notes

1 The information about the Carpenters was supplied by Dr William Cobb of Ridgewood, New Jersey, Mrs Carpenter's great grandson and Helena Carpenter Cobb's grandson, during a personal meeting in December 1994 at his house in Ridgewood.

2 Information gathered from the records of the Poughkeepsie Rural Cemetery where all the Carpenter children, with the exception of Viola, are buried in the Eighmie Lot.

3 Kanitkar, *Anandibai*, 2002, pp. 54–55.

4 *The Indian Ladies' Magazine*, Madras, January 1906, p. 210.

5 Kanitkar, *Anandibai*, 2002, pp. 55–57; my re-translation into English.

6 *Indian Ladies' Magazine*, January 1906, p. 210.

7 The letter is reproduced verbatim, with very minor editing, from a Xerox copy of the originals held in the Carpenter Family Archive.

8 *Indian Ladies' Magazine*, 1906, p. 210.

9 Ramabai Ranade, *Amachya Ayushyatil Kahi Athavani*, Pune: K. G. Sharangapani, 1953 (1910), p. 20; Athavale, p. 6; Tilak, p. 10; Anandibai Karve, Maze Puran, Ed. Kaveri Karve, 3rd ed., Bombay: Keshav Bhikaji Dhavale, 1998 (1944), p. 42.

10 By 'Banias' Anandibai probably means Jains.
11 Dall, p. 36.
12 Ibid.
13 Ibid.
14 Here Anandibai gives the mistaken impression that women formed parts of the procession. This was not so: all the women stayed at home.
15 Athavale, p. 7; Karve, p. 25.

3

AN INDO-AMERICAN
DIALOGUE

The act of letter-writing had rapidly become an enriching enough experience to prompt Anandibai to punctuality despite her recurrent illness, a cultural phenomenon qualitatively different from her earlier routine letters, enabling her to rediscover everyday life with fresh eyes.

Bhuj Post Office
15th November 1880

My dear sister,

My last letter was rather late on account of my illness. As I was again taken ill, I feared that I would not be able to mail this letter in time. But thanks be to Providence. He wills that we should be drawn closer and closer, and thus effect a union with ties which nothing can break. I am glad to say that I am much better now, and so proceed to answer your letter dated 1*st* September 1880 which remained unreplied last time.

When I received your letter for the first time, I had no taste for reading correspondence. Your second letter made me look to you for interesting matters and enabled me to see how daily occurrences of life which formerly were considered trifling were turned to account for instructing the mind. Your subsequent letters have opened my eyes to the contrast between the lives you and we lead. Whenever I was to write a letter to my friends and relations in India, I felt as if I had nothing to write upon, though surrounded by innumerable things for my amusement in literary pursuits. My eyes are now directed to the daily receipt of letters from you and my relations, and when they do not arrive in time when due, I am greatly disappointed, so much so that I do this at the sacrifice of my sleep and mental rest. This new tendency of mind is due to your generosity and good will towards others, for which I am exceedingly grateful

Anandibai's ambition for higher, especially medical studies, was periodically fuelled by this correspondence, despite the frustrating lack of opportunities in India.

It is my misfortune that we should be at such a distance from each other. When I feel that I should prosecute my studies more vigorously, I have not the means. I am more inclined to study medicine, but in vain. There are no schools or colleges, except [those] imparting rudimental knowledge to women. Alas! How unfortunate we are!

In the continuous discussion of Indian social customs, Anandibai displayed clear awareness of and reconciliation with the gendered double standards of morality, as well as the universal son preference in Indian families. It needs to be remembered that we have a fifteen-year-old girl writing these letters, albeit at a time when girls were compelled by circumstance to mature early.

We have no polygamy to speak of. Though there is no social or religious restriction [on] a man to marry as many times as he likes, yet the middle class [men] do not take more than one wife for fear that their coffer would be empty and they would run into debt from which they would never be extricated if once got into. The chiefs, princes, and generally higher classes have more than one wife. The Nizam of Hyderabad had 300 wives and the Sultan of Turkey in the West has as many now. Our people, if they at all take more than one wife, marry for the sake of sons if they do not have any by [the] first or second wife. So you see how fond we are of sons socially and religiously. The Heavens are open to the man who has a son but not otherwise. If a man dies without a son, his head is covered when his corpse is taken to the burning ground. There are many rites and funeral ceremonies which none but a son is eligible to perform and without which the dead [man] is supposed to be damned and hurled down to Hell.

From the reading matter to hand, especially the *Banner of Light*, I am led to believe that there are many ladies in America who are given to the study of spiritualism. There are many stories published in that paper to the effect that the dead appeared before the living and told many things to their survivors. Do you believe in them or are you an eye-witness to the manifestations? If so, please enlighten me.

Anandibai's interest in the occult surfaces here for the first time in this correspondence and was to continue. It was this interest, coupled with a nationalistic pride in India's 'glorious past', which seems to have led the Joshees to the newly established Theosophical Society.

I think you have heard of Madame Blavatsky and Colonel Olcott. They are making wonders in India. The papers are full [of] the account of the occult phenomena of Blavatsky. She is [a] staunch advocate of Vedic philosophy and asserts that all the new things discovered or invented were formerly in practice in India.

I do not expect much encouragement from the other members of my family. They are, properly speaking, orthodox to the letter, and cannot be expected to sympathise with me. But as my husband is so much in favour of . . . [giving women] emancipation, no one dares turn his face against me.

Anandibai's response to her situation is complex; her awareness of the social opposition to women's education has heightened her appreciation of her husband's courage, which protected her from this hostility. At the same time, exposed to the full blast of Orientalism and cherishing a desire for the superior benefits of Western education, she feels compelled to champion Hindu learning.

The Europeans are under the impression that there is nothing worth knowing in [the] Hindu scripture and I have therefore taken up *Sanscrit* [sic] to show them how sublime, useful and instructive are the precepts in Hindu Shastras. Should we meet, you see, I will be much benefitted. Your very letters convince me that you are an educated lady [at] whose feet I shall not be ashamed to sit.

Simultaneously there is Gopalrao's radical plan to send Anandibai alone to America for higher education provided it is financially viable and compatible with her (and perhaps also his) insistence on retaining the Brahmin way of life as much as possible.

My husband is greatly inclined to send me to America for the purpose of my being thoroughly instructed in some practical knowledge, but does not see his way to it. Suppose I come there with the intention of staying till I have passed one or two examinations, which will at least take more than three or four years. I am a vegetarian and do not wish to be Europeanised as regards my food and dress. Wherever I go, I wish to carry my manners and customs unless they are detrimental to my health. Do you . . . [think that I will be able to live] in your country in my own way? If so, what will be the monthly expense per head including school charges? I put these questions out of curiosity. It is not possible that I shall ever be so fortunate as to visit your land.

I intend going to my mother's for a month or so. My sister is very anxious to see me, so [are] my brother and mother, and I have been away from them these ten months. They have grown impatient.

My hearty and kind kisses to Eighmie and Helena for whom I send more flowers.

In return Anandibai also received dried flowers and leaves, and some serious literature.

Bhuj Post Office
15*th* December 1880

My dear sister,

I beg with many thanks to acknowledge receipt of your welcome and most interesting letter of 8*th* October 1880. I also thank you for the volume entitled *The History of the Origin of All Things* which came to hand together with three volumes of Maria King's work and other interesting matters, circulars and also very beautiful autumn leaves. I beg to offer my hearty thanks to Miss Amy Stewart for the kindness shown in sending me the picture of the house you live in. The house seems to be a very magnificent and princely one. It displays workmanship in its structure and position. I congratulate you upon having such a mansion surrounded by a beautiful garden. Please present my photo to Miss Amy Stewart.

As Mrs Carpenter's surroundings began to take shape through photos, Anandibai's circle of American friends began to widen. The Carpenters' neighbour, Ms Stewart, a potential friend and correspondent, and unusual for possessing a step-father, led Anandibai into a discussion of marriage customs in the two countries and their relative advantages.

I shall really be very happy if you will be pleased to ask Miss Amy Stewart to write me a letter. She must, no doubt, be a very accomplished lady. I am sorry she is fatherless. Among us there are many children who have a step-mother, but not a step-father; as you know widows in our caste are not allowed to marry again. Some reformers have introduced and are trying to introduce the remarriage system among the higher classes [i.e. castes]. Their object is to get these girls remarried who have lost their husbands before puberty. So you see there is none at present willing to marry a grown-up widow who has some children by her first husband. The reason is obvious. None likes to be burdened with another's children, while a woman does not grudge to marry a person who has children by his first wife as the onus of supporting them falls upon the latter. In many instances when step-children and step-mother do not pull on well, as is natural, the former are separated and the father lives together with his new wife, though at the same time he bears the expenses of both the houses. But in case a step-father does not have his step-children with him, where should they go and who should support them? [This] is the question which I hope you will kindly answer for my sake.

Anandibai's intellectual struggle between conventional and liberal ideas is transparent.

I do not know if you will like me [to] put you such questions. In the first place when I ponder over the subject of the connection between man and woman, I generally side with the so-called orthodox ideas. So long as woman is not on equal terms with man, it is better for her to be under certain social restrictions, such as 'not to marry again', ''to be subservient to man', 'to look upon her husband as God'. These are the enjoinments of our Shastras.

The operative clause here is 'so long as woman is not on equal terms with man'. In other words, the woman's subservient role as a husband-worshipping wife, being an imperative of the firmly entrenched Hindu patriarchy, is best observed through customs which reduce or eliminate her psychological tensions and conflicts. In short, women, handicapped with a lack of options, should consent to their own subordination. In the context of what follows, Anandibai's seeming anti-feminism appears essentially to be pragmatism, which then develops into a belief in ultimate gender equality, to be achieved through Western influence and individual self-reliance, and further, to a nationalistic exposé of the reverse side of European society – the same society which is held as a role model for educated Indians.

> On the other hand, when I think over the sufferings to which woman is [subjected] in all ages and at all times, I grow impatient to see the Western light dawn upon us as the harbinger of emancipation and future good. Here I feel my inability to express myself as fully as I think. I am led to believe that man and woman should be self-protecting and that one should not depend upon the other for maintenance and other necessaries of life. Then and only then, family discord and social humiliation will cease completely. I am very sorry to see that there are many ladies among Europeans in India who are educated and accomplished for the purpose of marriage. Alas! How mischievous it is for a lady to adorn [herself] and change [her] dress every hour in order to allure bachelors.

Suddenly, Anandibai veers towards household composition, presenting the picture of a happy, harmonious extended family as typical of India (which she was to retract in a subsequent letter) – a trend of thought obviously triggered by the information of Amy Stewart's mother and step-father, Mr and Mrs Andrus, who were close to the Carpenters (and possibly shared parts of the same house).

> I am glad to hear that your family and that of Mr and Mrs Andrus are a very happy household. Indians are world-renowned for such happy households. There are many many [sic] families in which 10 or 12 brothers with their wives and children live together in one house from generation to generation. There are some houses the members of which number above 100. They all dine together, household affairs being divided and allotted to each female member. Is it not a marvel?

Anandibai's obvious exaggeration in sketching a large, idyllic family is surprising because of her usually honest and realistic assessment of Indian families and society. That there was a fair amount of friction and subjection of young daughters-in-law to coercive behaviour comes across vividly in the autobiographical narratives of her contemporary Brahmin women, such as Ramabai Ranade and Kashibai Kanitkar.[1]

Mrs Carpenter's keenness to meet Anandibai halfway in their friendship obviously led to questions about her life and country (and comparisons with other Asian countries, in this case, Burma, now Myanmar) which could be construed as inquisitive and perhaps offensive. Anandibai hastened to put her at her ease on this score ('I am always at your service. . . . Any questions you ask will be promptly replied to') and reiterated that it was such a privilege to receive letters from her, and she was 'ever ready to serve you with all my heart and soul'.

Anandibai then proceeds to describe that the Indian   houses are 'large and commodious as your bungalows', but not elegant, nor furnished with chairs, tables, or cots. The walls and floor were swept daily and smeared with cow-dung every week. (One wonders what Mrs Carpenter made of this.) Then comes a description of mattresses, pillows, and blankets of various thicknesses for the different seasons. Each person required a (metal) plate for bread (earlier she had spoken of banana leaves used as plates) and a couple of bowls for curried vegetables. One ate with one's fingers, without knives, forks, and spoons. Usually all men and young girls ate first, and were served by older women, who ate last. Anandibai's description of men's and women's dress is even more sketchy and inadequate. She is not able to properly describe men's *dhotar*, or lower garment, which is tied around the waist, with pleats tucked in, and the central hem passed between the legs to be tucked in at the back so that both legs are separately sheathed. They usually covered their upper body with another long piece of cloth at home, except in the hot season. For outdoor wear they put on a shirt (*angarkha*) tied across the chest with thin strips of cotton (which she omits altogether). A woman's sari, almost nine yards, was worn the same way, but then the remaining portion was swept up along the left shoulder to cover the bosom and brought forward to cover the right shoulder and upper arm as well. Then comes an account of the 'ritual pure' clothes worn during meals. The habit of chewing betel nuts among older women and eating the betel leaf prepared with the nut and other special ingredients (*vida* or *paan*) after meals among younger men and women is then described. No vices existed among Brahmins, she claimed, except for the newfangled one of drinking liquor among men. Then follows a description of various types of teeth-cleaning devices in different regions, from half-burnt cow-dung to snuff, to small (*neem*) twigs chewed into a brush at one end.

The payment of the books sent by Mrs Carpenter was next discussed, and then the interesting account of American national holidays and the presidential election. The letter was accompanied by a silver pen holder, a thimble, and 'specimens of Cutch work' for Eighmie.

*

The beginning of 1881 found Anandibai on a visit to her parental home in Kalyan, for a change of scenery and rest. The fifteen-year-old Anandibai and her younger brother Vinayak had to accomplish it without a proper escort. Gopalrao had taken them to Bhuj harbour, pointed out the steamer, and left them to fight their way through the crowds to board it. Fortunately, they met Mrs Batty, who was going by the same steamer to Mumbai. When chided by an acquaintance who witnessed the incident for his uncaring ways, Gopalrao merely shrugged the whole thing off.

Anandibai celebrated the festival of Makar Sankranti with her parents at Kalyan and sent the customary *tilgul* (sesame seeds coated with jaggery or sugar) to Mrs Carpenter in a silver box, along with other silver articles for which Bhuj was famous. By this time the requested photo of the motherly Mrs Carpenter had arrived, inspiring even greater affection in Anandibai.

Kalyan
20*th* January 1881

My dear sister,
    In your last letter was found enclosed what I longed to see, i.e., a picture of one who is my hope and pride, prized above all prizes; it is the portrait of her on whom rests my ambition, it is the likeness of one whose mind and soul are bent upon doing good to such creatures of God as are sincere searchers of truth and knowledge. I regret my inability to do justice to it in [the] terms you deserve. I can, however, say this much, that you rank next to none but my great Rishis and sages of old whose religion was truth, charity and austerity and who thereby attained eternal felicity. You seem to be resigned and satisfied with all in this world. Your reading is deep and your learning is vast and [both] are portrayed on your countenance. Good will and kind nature are visible in the picture in which you stand and look. Your face is full of love and so charming that I have often stood looking at it for hours together. This description is no exaggeration on my part but has been certified to be correct by many whom I had the pleasure of shewing your photo. Your picture before me leads me to believe that you have the knowledge of the past and future, and can discern what is going on in my mind, though at a considerable distance. If it is so as it should be, I need not say how full is my heart with respect, reverence and affection for you and [your] children. I am quite

sure that it is your power to know one's heart which led you to write to me first. You may have come across my husband's letter to Mr Wilder in America but that [cannot] be [a] sufficient reason to induce you to be kind and loving to me, better than my own relatives. If I am wrong please correct me. We are day by day being tied closely and firmly, and I have no doubt that in a short time we shall [become] one in feeling and dealing. I already wish and feel that I should call you my aunt. There is a saying among us, 'it does not matter much if a mother dies, but let not an aunt die'. This expression will show you in what respect and estimation a maternal aunt is held among us. If you allow me, I wish to look upon you as such.

Anandibai's wish to legitimise her friendship with Mrs Carpenter in terms of a surrogate relationship was very typically Indian. In 1883 Pandita Ramabai addressed her elderly spiritual guide Sister Geraldine of the Community of St Mary the Virgin at Wantage, England, as 'dear old Ajeebai', literally 'dear venerable grandmother', possibly because her little daughter addressed her as such.[2] Anandibai's letter then continues with a detailed description of the typical Maharashtrian celebration of Makar Sankranti.

As Mrs Carpenter's reply arrived during Anandibai's prolonged visit to Kalyan, Gopalrao took the opportunity to write a short letter to Mr Carpenter, combining the proper degree of formality with a hint at common intellectual interests and the richness of Indian spiritual literature.

> Bhuj Post Office
> 20th February [1881]

Dear Sir,

Allow me to address you. I have perused with interest the correspondence between my wife and Mrs Carpenter, and beg to ask you to thank her on my behalf for all the troubles taken and interest and care shown towards my wife . . .

I have read some portions of the *History of the Origin of All Things* so kindly presented to my wife by Mrs Carpenter. It is very easy in style but so difficult to understand that it no doubt requires to be studied prayerfully as Mrs Carpenter writes to say. I am glad both of you take such a lively interest in the study of mind and soul, but how important would it be to you to study Vedic literature in the East on the same subject?

As this is the first time I have had the pleasure of addressing you, though your name has been a family [i.e. household] word ever since the correspondence was opened with my wife by the kindness & all love of Mrs Carpenter, I shall not be justified in writing you a long letter. So I conclude with hearty regards for Mrs Carpenter and self, and kind kisses and love to children.

Yours sincerely
G.V. Joshee

Anandibai's own letter followed in March 1881, with apologies and a reference to her now chronic illness.

[Nasik?]
Bombay Presidency
March 81

My dearest sister,

I am exceedingly sorry that I was not able to send you my usual letter during . . . February. I beg to apologise for it, as it was partly owing [to] my illness and partly owing to . . . [family matters which forced me to come to Poona] . . .

I am sorry I am taken ill so often. But I assure you I shall never stop writing to you [perhaps not] punctually but positively certainly. It is the will of God and heavenly spirits that we should be drawn closer and closer, and I hope that I shall never cease to be what I should be. Your letters are full of interesting and instructive matters and are a treat to me. I pray to God to give you [a] long life and enable you to accomplish your noble aims and fulfil your desires.

I am really astonished to see that you have no faith in the present doctors. Our [case] is the reverse. We commit ourselves to the doctor's care implicitly. We never question his ability and curative powers. Your letter leads [one] to suppose that there are more than enough doctors in America, nay, medical knowledge must be so widely spread that every man and woman is constituted his or her own doctor. It is then quite possible that you have no confidence in anybody's prescription. This is as it should be. But our case is quite different. In India medical advice is so expensive & rare that thousands upon thousands depend upon nature for cure. All diseases . . . arise from indigestion. When we are rather indisposed, fasting is at once resorted to. In Benares where the atmosphere is very thick, and digestive power generally deranged, persons suffering from fever abstain from food and drink for 21 days, sometimes 40. This is no exaggeration.

The mention of illness naturally led to a long, drawn-out discussion about the effects of child marriage. Surprisingly, Anandibai is almost aggressive in her insistence that women's health problems arose not solely or even primarily from child marriage, but either from the institution of marriage itself or from independent causes which affected even unmarried women, because European women also suffered from similar complaints. Throughout her correspondence Anandibai uses terms like 'civilised countries' and 'Natives', as was common in the Indo-British or even Indian discourse.

> Early marriage is no doubt a bane. When we deviate from the laws of nature, we must suffer the consequences. The practice of early marriage is not prevalent in many countries and yet the women there often are weak and ill-constituted as we are. I know of one lady (who was a spinster) who was always complaining of some thing or the other, and never appeared in good health. So there [are] many European ladies in India, old and young, whose faces are pale and gloomy. There is no bloom on their countenances. I do not know the cause. If it is early marriage, as many of us suppose, I shall feel obliged if you will kindly account for the same condition perceptible in all civilised countries [in] which there is . . . no early marriage. Early marriage will no doubt be one of the causes which lead to this havoc and destruction of life. I admit that the condition of Indian women is miserable and deplorable. . . . [But it would be undesirable] if we . . . destroy all the old institutions as pernicious without having something better to substitute [for] them. [The] European mode of life and delicacy of manners and customs are not appreciable as they appear on the very face, expensive, and not within the reach of the masses. Anything that cannot be enjoyed by the masses must be bad. I, however, hope that you will kindly enlighten me on [the] subject I have so rudely and without regard to logic or reasoning handled above. My defence of our present customs and manners will at least show you how ignorant we are and how prejudiced are our opinions about anything that is now [prevalent].

Surprisingly, Mrs Carpenter seems to have supported early, though not prepubertal, marriage, and was possibly under the mistaken impression that Hindu marriages were consummated before puberty.

> You say that Nature has designed us to mate at an early age and therefore infer that we must be married early but not before puberty. If this be the cause why we women . . .[?] earlier, our people would not have brought so much pressure to bear against widow remarriage, but it is neither Nature nor religion to blame for introducing early marriage. There must be something else which I leave up to you to solve.

Mrs Carpenter's concern for Anandibai had led her to inquire after her fate in case of possible widowhood, and to suggest means of bypassing the ordeals faced by the internally troped Hindu widow. Anandibai discusses the matter candidly and dispassionately, conveying her resignation to custom and social pressure for the sake of her family, as well as illustrating the dilemma of all her contemporary reformers caught between progressive ideas which propelled them forward and ties of blood which often pulled them back.

> Should it be my misfortune to survive my husband, [though] God and custom forbid me to have such an idea, I should have no other alternative but to submit to fate and the humiliation and degradation which falls to the lot of widows. As long as I wish to be dutiful to my mother and loving to my brother and sister, and pleasant to all my other nearest relatives, I cannot but act as their loving tenderness dictates.

Just this one sentence brings out the helplessness of a person in that social milieu which made even ties of affection contingent upon conforming to a rigid gendered social code.

> No written will or decree from my husband will turn the tide and current of fate in any other direction and *will me a whit better* (?) unless I resolve to act otherwise than they wish. When overwhelmed with grief and sorrow, and surrounded by none but those merciless and stone hearted creatures, let it be my mother, father or sisters, I do not think I shall have the presence of mind to resist their wishes. My husband's will or decree will then be of no avail. I do not understand what you mean

when you urge us both to move out of the reach of Brahmins. If you wish that we should embrace any other religion, and thus sever our connection with society, it will be equally difficult, perhaps harder. In both cases I will expose myself to the ridicule and general condemnation which rends hardy hearts. The misery will abate, the custom will change as civilization and progress advance but the thought that many will be crushed down before the time of the release from the shackles arrives, is painful to me. Dear sister, I am so thankful to you for the anxiety and sisterly care you bear for me. The fact that I have a kind and dear friend in you to sympathise with me in all my afflictions is more than encouraging and soothing, and will enable me to bear with resignation and fortitude the vicissitudes of life. I am quite at a loss to convey in fitting terms the warmth of affection and gratefulness I feel towards you. Dear and benevolent sister, the idea of bereavement as you have mooted and touched upon in your letter has made me uneasy and restless.

In this connection Anandibai again dwells upon the double standards of morality embedded in the Hindu sacred books, and reveals her own gender-egalitarian beliefs. Significantly, she tries to reinforce them with mythological ('historical') stories as evidence.

Men and women are saved alike by good and meritorious actions, but the duties prescribed to obtain the end [salvation] are different [in Hinduism]. Like [among] the Mormons, husbands are the altar on which women should make the sacrifice of self, in other words, they should worship husband as God. There is no other duty enjoined for the salvation of women. But I do not believe so. I am warranted [guaranteed?] by the shastras that man and woman attain eternal bliss by [the] same deeds. It is no doubt perverted imagination [and] false traditions that dictate that man should do one thing and woman the other. . . .

In ancient times women were versed in astronomy and all other sciences. So we are not like [the] Chinese or Mahommedans, but [the] flow of circumstances has reduced us to this state of degradation from which none but the Almighty can rescue us.

Again the pride of the 'glorious past' of the Hindus, whom Anandibai consistently projects as superior to other Asians, is evident. One idea current at the time was that the ancient Hindu wisdom, which predated learning in other countries, was diffused in historical times successively to Egypt, the Roman Empire, and then on to England. But while all these countries increased this wisdom several-fold, the Hindus themselves lost it completely; hence their present degeneracy.[3]

> I have already sent the nose ring as promised. I hope you have received it. I have also sent some sugar-mixed seeds to be distributed among children and others.[4]
>
> Many thanks for the samples of Miss Stewart's dress and of your black satin de Lyon. I think the cloth is oily as the paper was spoilt by their colour. Please give my respects to your stepmother and husband, and love and kisses to children.[5] I beg to acknowledge receipt of your favour dated *6th* January 81 with New Year cards. Please accept my thanks for the same and tell Miss Stewart that I am so much obliged by the kindness shown me in many respects. I am so glad that both of you are interested in India and Indian women. The cards are beautifully decorated and varied in design. I am sorry that I have not got any such things to send you in return. So accept my thanks in return. . . .
>
> Yours affectionately
Anandibai Joshee

Notes

1 Ranade, *Amachya Ayushyatil*; Vaidya, *Shrimati Kashibai.*
2 *The Letters and Correspondence of Pandita Ramabai.*
3 *The Letters and Correspondence of Pandita Ramabai*, p. 285.
4 The reference seems to be to *tilgul*, a sweet made of sesame seeds and jaggery, distributed among relatives and friends during the days following 'Makar Sankranti' (about the middle of January). March is too late for this, but Anandibai had missed the February letter.
5 There is no reference to Mrs Carpenter having had a stepmother. Her father Jeremiah Eighmie (1810–1895) and mother Naomie Jane Eighmie (1830–1904) are buried in the Eighmie Lot of the Poughkeepsie Rural Cemetery.

4

THE BENGAL INTERLUDE
Calcutta

Soon afterwards, Gopalrao obtained a transfer to Calcutta (now Kolkata) through his prior acquaintance with Mr James, Post Master General of Calcutta. Gopalrao had been motivated by the news that the postal department of the Bengal Presidency offered jobs to women. His new ambition – again centering vicariously on his wife – visualised Anandibai as being among the first batch of these working women. He came increasingly to rely on her as a means of making his mark in the world. Full of these ambitious plans he joined his new duties on 6 April 1881.

But the move from western to eastern India meant crossing over into a new world – geographically, culturally, and linguistically. The fertile, textile-rich, and commercially developed eastern India had been the earliest British territorial acquisition in the Indian subcontinent, dating from the mid-eighteenth century. The power centre of the Presidency and the capital of British India was the port-city of Calcutta on the Hooghly River, about eighty miles north of the Bay of Bengal. It enjoyed the same urban predominance in the area as Mumbai did in western India.

As the seat of the Viceroy of India, as well as the Lieutenant-General of the Bengal Presidency, Calcutta ranked high within the British Empire. In addition to administrative, maritime, and commercial functions, it was at the forefront of new reformist socio-religious movements. As the cradle of the Indian renaissance, Bengal and Calcutta enjoyed a nationwide leadership role, although the binary between a few reformers and the majority of conservative anti-reformers remained here as well.

The Joshees unfortunately seem to have been singularly unlucky in their initial exposure to this new socio-cultural milieu. Their arrival was promptly reported to Mrs Carpenter in April 1881:

> My dearest sister,
>   We arrived here on the 4*th* and I had no time to write as promised in my last, on account of [the] unexpected transfer,

but I now sit down to answer your letter dated 23rd January 1881 which was simultaneously received with that preceding it. I have yet two more letters to reply to, which came to hand a few days ago. I will try to answer these also in the course of this month. So you will have three letters from me this month. . . .

I am very glad to see that the articles I sent have contributed so much to the pleasure and delight of my American little darlings, whose charming photos are hung in my bedroom/ sleeping room, and whom I am so anxious to embrace and kiss personally. I will try to send them some specimens of Cutchi needle work. I shall be exceedingly happy to have a letter in their own handwriting.

The flowers that I sent you were not of the best sort, but wild ones. I had made a little garden in my compound at Bhuj. I had no liking for such innocent and charming sceneries! But I owe you an immense debt for cultivating in me the habit of flower-planting. As a rule, we are not fond of flowers as a personal pleasure. Our religious men and women get up early in the morning and go to the nearest garden of their own or of anybody else, and gather lots of flowers, not for personal use or for adorning houses and tables, but to worship God therewith. They do not smell them, nor do they allow children to come near or to touch them. Any flower spoilt by children or fallen on the trodden ground, or smelt by anyone, becomes unfit for the purpose of worship. The best of flowers are consecrated to the service of Gods. . . .

Anandibai's fervent wish to enlarge her circle of American friends remained unfulfilled, though she continued to hope for a letter from the elusive Ms Stewart. She looked at her American pen-friends as a source of enlightenment on various subjects earlier outside her ken. But perhaps the openness of these communications, not possible within the rigid and closed relationships within the Indian family, appealed to her. Perhaps they helped keep alive her slender hope of going to America.

I am very thankful to Miss Stewart for her willingness to favour me with a letter. When she writes, I will have two ladies in America whom I can reckon among the best friends of mine and well-wishers. My power of keeping correspondence with you both will then increase and I will thus be educated by 'post'.

The old discussion about child marriage was now revived, and Anandibai's vacillation ended somewhat abruptly with an explicit and radical statement endorsing British legislation for introducing social reform:

> We have many societies for the prevention of early marriage, but they cannot exercise [a] powerful influence over the irresistible tendencies of the generality of people. Almost all the rich and influential people are orthodox to the letter and cannot be prevailed upon to put a stop to heinous customs and manners unless the strong ruling force interferes. The custom of 'suttee' has been forcibly abolished and the early marriage [custom] requires a similarly deadly blow before it can give way.

In the same candid manner Anandibai explodes the myth of the happy and harmonious extended family – a myth she has herself built up in an earlier letter.

> It is no wonder to us that so many brothers harmoniously live together. It is not because the system is advantageous that so many live together, but because separation is a crime socially and religiously. If a man cannot put up with and bear, with resignation, the family inconveniences, he is pronounced to be unfit for higher spheres of life. I do not know how far this theory is correct, but I give it out as it is current.

A view gaining currency among reformers was that Indians were lazy and lacked industriousness, and had only themselves to blame for their poverty. About a year later, in June 1882, Pandita Ramabai published the Marathi book *Stri Dharma Niti*, in which she dwelt upon this point at length, commenting that the present dependent and wretched condition of her people was due to lack of diligence.[1] In the same vein Anandibai writes:

> I find fault with my countrymen and women, because they are so indolent. The best artists in India are very near starving, for they do not want work; the poorest people are quite contented with bare bread if they get it for nothing. There are thousands upon thousands of beggars who are half clothed and half fed, and yet live on public charity. The working population of India is outnumbered by begging one in the ratio of one to 100. It is therefore no wonder that the country is impoverished and

degenerated. I do not know when we will be a busy body [!] like yours. It is pleasant to work as it leaves no room for idle speculation. Why should you then complain of the constant strain on the nervous system? The laws of Nature are unfathomable. Sloth lacks industry while the latter pines for the former.

Underlying Anandibai's affection and regard for Mrs Carpenter was a deep feeling of gratitude which led her to regard the latter as a great soul sent to Earth to save mankind – an idea echoing the famous description of Krishna in the *Bhagavad Gita*, as one who appears on Earth in human guise to protect the good and destroy the wicked.

You are indeed far superior in intellect and learning. You are a lady of deep erudition. I will not be worth the lacenet [?] of your shoes. I feel shame when I see you scale me so high. Had it not been for your generous heart which prompted you to cast on me your benevolent eye, I would not have felt the darkness in which I am groping. If it be the will of God to ever raise me to the level of my fortunate sisters in the civilised countries, it will be through the aid and countenance of you and suchlike philanthropists whose existence in this world is for the good of others. God has from time to time sent down on earth magnanimous persons to save mankind. I look upon you as such. . . .

My letter has already been too long and I therefore beg to conclude with love and kisses to children and regards for self and husband. . . .

Yours affectionately
Anandibai Joshee

*

The couple's move to Bengal turned out to be a major upheaval, with various unhappy experiences in Calcutta. The hot and humid climate considerably aggravated Anandibai's chronic health problems. The Bengali social milieu caused a culture shock. The neighbours were unfriendly and the couple's progressive behaviour scandalised not only the more strictly gender-segregated Bengali society, but also the Europeans who had come to accept it as the Indian norm. Worst of all, the Joshees' household goods were delayed in transit, which made even the daily cooking a problem in view of the strict rules of ritual purity which required only a certain type of metal pot and prohibited the intake of food cooked by anyone but a Maharashtrian Brahmin.

In her very next letter, 9 May 1881, Anandibai poured out her tale of woe to Mrs Carpenter, albeit with a characteristic philosophical touch. But the debate on social matters continued.

> My dear sister,
> . . . I am also disposed to think in the manner you do that true conjugal love cannot be divided without loss. But example is better than precept. We have many instances in India indicating that the love of many [multiple] wives for their one husband is as good as that of one husband and one wife. . . . I know of many cases in which the husbands are vicious and profligate and their wives are so faithful that they are ready to burn themselves on the [funeral] pyres of their husbands should they die. If, as you say, the love is divided, how will you account for such rare virtue adorning many a heart in India? In civilised countries polygamy is not sanctioned by the Church and the law. But where is the security for pure life? It is in the mouths of many sincere Englishmen. This nation [England?] is corrupt and has no moral bindings. There are many women there in England who indulge secretly before they are married and are yet eligible for marriage. We have no such instances in India as we marry before we know what it is for. I do not mean to say that there are not bad women among the married ones, but human nature is just the same all over the world. But there is this advantage in early marriage that the husband marries a pure and chaste girl. In grown-up marriages no such confidence can be attained. It would be very difficult for my husband to know what I do behind [his back] and vice versa, beyond conjecturing which is not always correct. Many innocent lives are put to death on false charges. I cannot therefore say whether polygamy or monogamy is congenial to the happy growth.

Anandibai's ingrained *pativrata* ideal surfaces here again in full force, as does the contrast between the pure Indian woman and the morally suspect Western woman. Her thoughts turn to the Hindu belief that a son alone can save the parents from going to hell after death (by performing the requisite rituals), and then to the occult communion with the dead, which seems to have interested Mrs Carpenter deeply as well.

> We have no faith in [the] saving influence of a son, but we have no messages from the dead. I have lost my son, father, mother, and sisters, but cannot realise their existence & happy life in

heaven. I wish I had that pleasure of communicating with and hearing from my relatives. I look forward to the time when you will initiate me into the mysteries of Nature.

We are very thankful to you and your medical friend for all the hopes and promises held out to us. It is indeed very kind of you to take so much interest in me, I really wish that I should see you and thus enjoy the blessings you are so ready to confer on me, but it is idle to suppose that I shall ever be so fortunate as to be able to undertake a journey to a distant country.

The feeling of depression and gloom was rooted in a series of disheartening experiences in Calcutta, resulting from culture shock, alienation, and loneliness, exacerbated by an unpleasant and possibly racially prejudiced European landlady. The 'misfortune' which threatened Gopalrao's job is explained in another letter.

Before I came to Calcutta, I had hopes but they are all vanished. We have been overtaken by so many misfortunes that I do not think my husband will continue long in the service. We no doubt came here for good but our stars are bad and will not let us prosper. We have no friends here; our diet, manners, and customs are different from those of the Bengalis, the inhabitants of this country. Even we could not claim the sympathy of the English. Here is a milliner in whose house we live. She is such a bad and cruel lady that she tried her best to disturb us. When I came here, all her servants gathered around me just to have a look at me. The lady also began to peep through her windows and to laugh in her sleeve. If we sat reading [aloud], she would send us a word not to read as her children cannot go to sleep. She got up stories. Once she gave it out that we are not pulling [on] well with each other and then she spread a rumour that we quarrelled the whole night, so much so that the other tenants were awakened. This did not satisfy her. She then gave it out that I am not a married woman but [a] kept one. This sort of treatment from a German lady towards perfect strangers must be disturbing & heart-rending. For a fortnight or so, we could not get enough to eat though our pocket was full. Our kit baggage, bedding, & clothing all remained behind and we had to content ourselves with mats to sleep on. The floor or ground was so damp that the few clothes we had on became wet, and we felt chilly. Such a time had never befallen us before. This will show you how hard it is to travel in countries where we have no friends to comfort us. What then will be our condition in a country where everything is strange?

It now becomes apparent that Gopalrao was apt to lose his head in an emergency such as this, and that it was Anandibai who kept a level head and gave him courage.

My husband has therefore given up all hope. He says now, that it is no use being forward in the face of so many difficulties resulting from going away from the trodden path of the society amongst which we live. But I . . . tell him to have courage . . . this is a trial and we must not lose spirit. This world is full of hardships and sufferings.

. . . I also send you the railway map of India from which you will please see where I was before and where I am now.

I cannot write more as I am suffering from boils. I will give some account in my next letter of my travels & the places I have visited.

With love and kisses to children, and kind regards to self and husband.

I remain

Yours very affectionately
Anandibai Joshee

The situation did not improve on any front, resulting in a deepening depression. The culture shock brought the realisation that if travel within India was so fraught with obstacles, the ambition to visit alien shores was too unrealistic to cherish. This inner turmoil was shared with Mrs Carpenter in the letter of June 1881. Anandibai's health problems and mental depression led her thoughts repeatedly to death, or perhaps a premonition of death. One of the few redeeming features she clung to was her strong and intensely affectionate friendship with Mrs Carpenter – now her 'aunt' – to the extent of finding American remedies for her illness. In June 1881 she wrote

My dear Aunt,

Though words are words and we are all flesh and blood, yet we are not satisfied with the nakedness with which we come down on earth. As clothes are made to hide indecency, so words are made to express the relation in which we stand to each other. When I proposed to call you by this name ['Aunt'], I was not sure you would accord your consent to it, but your willingness to allow me to indulge in my own way is a sign which augurs well for the future; I have now the pleasure to console myself that I am more under care and kindness, and [that] you will not forget me.

I am really sorry that I should be so unfortunate as to be unable to satisfy the longing for my letters so kindly evinced in your last. As I told you before, Calcutta is trying us to the utmost. Physically we are so reduced in strength and health, that we cannot digest the food taken in the morning till the next day. The climate is awfully warm and I am fearfully suffering from boils. My face has a thousand gettings up which had made me so hideous. It has commenced raining, and yet the heat is not less. I do not know how long we have to continue in this miserable state.

. . . I have always something to complain of. Sometimes I am so uneasy and restless that I feel hardly able to speak or breathe. This comes upon me so frequently that I do not think that I shall live long. Sometimes life is a burden. My husband comes home fatigued and tired, and goes to sleep as soon as he has his back on the bed, while I lie by his side sleepless for hours together. I wish that he should speak with me till I am able to shut my eyes, but he cannot do so for which I am always angry with him, though it is not his fault. Headache & fever are my common complaints. I therefore candidly ask you to recommend me to your kind Doctor and let me know what he says. Any change in climate makes me uneasy. Your country would suit me best. I ask my husband to start for America as India would do us no good.

This drastic step seemed to have been dictated by the suffocating atmosphere of Calcutta's strictly gender-segregated society:

There are people here who would never let us alone. We go out for a walk in the evening, and European ladies and gentlemen are wonderstruck at it and keep [looking] at us from a distance till we or they go out of sight. They point to us and seem [to talk] about us. The case is still more striking with the natives. They come to a standstill when they see us pass by. They would not move an inch. I have observed some natives in carriages to order their coachmen to stop when they come near us, and not drive [on] till their curiosity is gratified. The people around us have such misgivings that they can never be persuaded to believe that we are married. The reason is not far to seek. There is so much of [the] zenana system in this part of the country, that a woman can scarcely stand in [the] presence of her own relations, [far] less in [the] presence of her husband.[2] Her face is always veiled, and she is not allowed to speak with any man. . . . there is a peculiar way of conveying modesty about us; in the absence of which we can but pass for something else. Even the Babus who [have] spent some years in England and America cannot walk or drive in the company of their wives in open carriages. If you go to their houses, you will see zenana too rigidly observed. If it is so with the educated people, how much more prejudiced must then be illiterate ones. One Police Sepoy had once the impudence to come near us when taking a walk in the Esplanade and ask my husband who this woman was with him. This irritated my husband and he had to ask the person's name in order to report him to the commissioner. This brought him to [his] senses and he left us alone after exchanging courtesies. All this naturally leads me to conclude that either this country is not good for us, or we are behaving in a manner unwarranted by the customs of this country. If the former conclusion is correct, I am not then wrong in pressing my husband to get out of it, but he says it would be rashness on our part were we to go to a foreign land, uncared for and unprotected.

The depression renewed Anandibai's interest in the occult, and she pressed Mrs Carpenter for details of her experiences. The letter ends with her usual expression of affection and regard.

This was followed by a postcard dated 23 July 1881:

My dear Aunt,

I am very sorry to say that I am insuperably [?] suffering from boils and I cannot sit to write a letter. I have yet three letters to answer but I am compelled to postpone them to next Saturday. I received a letter from Eighmie enclosed in your last. I was very glad to read it. Little Eighmie writes very well. I hope she will continue responding without fail. . . . Many many thanks for [the] piece of ribbon sent by her. I keep it in my favourite book, with great alacrity. The inclemency of [the] weather is now less as it has commenced to rain and we both are now better.

The next letter was dated 6 August 1881:

My dear Aunt,

. . . I had promised to give a reply last Saturday, as I did not do so, you perhaps will not believe in me as a true niece. But I have the [best] excuse in my business, as we are removing from this house to another. . . .

Next comes a glowing account of the life-style of a holy Brahmin, followed by personal matters.

I was very glad to hear that Mrs Andrus gave birth to a daughter and both mother and child were doing well. It is the custom among us that when we hear of the birth [among] our relations or friends, we send them dresses for the child and its mother. . . . Ten days [the mother and child] are supposed to be unclean. . . . On the twelfth day all the friends and relations are invited together for a feast. . . . Then the child is put in a cradle and named with great joy. And then it is rocked by the women gathered around, who sing [a] good many songs about God. Is there anything like this in America?

In Anandibai's letter of 17 August, the dialogue reverted to married life, its potential oppressiveness for Indian women, the misery of Indian widowhood, and Mrs Carpenter's fear of such a fate befalling Anandibai:

You have correctly detailed the circumstances which enfeeble women. I agree with you in the main. It should be the motto of men and women to live independent of each other. One should not be housed for the other, then half of the miseries of this world will be alleviated. Don't suppose even for a moment that the peace of my mind was disturbed by your inquiries as to how I would fare in the event of [my] husband's death. I was on the contrary very glad to answer your sympathetic queries. I do not share the old prejudices, nor do I give much weight to old customs and manners, but mentioned them for your information. You should take them as not applicable to me. We are both growing fast in new tenets and principles. We have chalked out our path of life quite differently from that of our ancestors, but cannot fully work it out for many constitutional and social difficulties. Soon after my marriage, or say [even] before that, my husband got my parents bound to give their tacit consent to my future education in any way he liked. His object . . . was the same as you cared for. That I may not be subjected to social degradation and humiliation, and lead the life more of a slave than of an intelligent being after his death, he set aside all religious and social restrictions and sent me to school in spite of all opposition. He will not be satisfied till I shall be able to live as you wish me to. So you need not be saddened. All that my heart longs for is that I should be near you, so that I may be beyond the limits of arbitrary customs. I thank you for your kind wishes that we should be drawn closer and closer & that God and angels shall bless the friendship thus singularly begun.

. . . I am very much obliged to Mrs Andrus' Irish cook for the tract sent by her. I have read it and found it very useful and instructive. I wish I had many such kind-hearted and devout souls around me.

Eighmie's letter was acknowledged with pleasure and compliments, and a length of gold-bordered silk for a dress promised to her.

I have already given you some descriptions of the Indian railway carriages. I have no doubt enjoyed a variety and beauty of scenery along the route. From Bombay to Bhosawal, the country is mountainous and not attractive, but . . . [beyond] you find the country flat bordering on the horizon. The plains are very fertile and productive of all grain. It is interspersed by many large rivers, some of which are two or three miles wide. In this part of the country, there are many important towns and cities of historical note, of which there would be very few in Europe who have not heard, such as Laknow [Lucknow], Kanpur, Jhansee [Jhansi], Agra, Gwalior, etc. in my future letters I will try to give an account of all the stations I have visited.

I beg to congratulate you upon Roselle being the centre and terminus of so many trains. Kalyan where I have been in December last, is [a] junction station through which all the trains from north and south have to pass before they go to and from Bombay, but the number of trains is not so large as 130. The reason is that [not many people travel by train].

My husband asks me to communicate his best thanks to Mr Carpenter for the elaborate letter he was pleased to send him. My husband will take the earliest opportunity to write him a thanks-giving letter. . . .

If you see or write to your mother again, please convey my best regards to her and also to your venerable father and brother. I wish I could see them all.

We have many artificial flowers for sale in the market, but we never make use of them for dresses, nor do we put them on hats or bonnets.

We are removed from Park Street. Please therefore to direct (your letters) to the care of the General Post Office as before. Our stay in Calcutta is uncertain, and as we are involved in ever growing anxieties as to our future destiny, I do not know now to what direction the stream of events will run. At all events, we shall not retract our steps to where we came from. Our motto will, in future, be 'Forward'.

Before the Joshees recovered from these troubles, a new and more terrible blow fell. Gopalrao inadvertently lost a very important dispatch from the Viceroy, and was immediately suspected of treason. Anandibai wrote the following on 27 August 1881:

My dear Aunt,

. . . Your letter I am about to reply to is so consoling and heart soothing and so [timely?] that it is a welcome one.

We are not yet free from troubles. During the period of the last five months, we had anxieties arising from without and within. We were about to forget them, when another serious mishap occurred. A special dispatch from the Viceroy to the Governor of Bengal was due here on Sunday, the 14th. It was watched by special officers from Simla.[3] It was received at Calcutta by my husband on passing a receipt. It was to be immediately sent to the Governor's camp. My husband was therefore going to the railway station with one of his assistants, into whose hands the important letter was given. As they were running fast to get into a hackney carriage that could be met on the road . . . the letter dropped down within the distance of one-eighth of a mile. A searching inquiry was made all along the road, but in vain. The letter disappeared in the twinkling of an eye. The consternation and stir it must have given rise to throughout the town will be the better conceived than described. All the high officials held counsel. The police were sent in all directions. The persons of the men on the road were examined, and not a stone was left unturned. My husband and his assistants were in police custody. Depositions were drawn before each officer. In short, it was a day which shall never be forgotten. My husband was suspended pending orders from Government.

You may imagine what state of mind I must have been in, and how engrossed my heart must have been by grief! We gave up all hopes of service, and were preparing to start for any place in view. We first determined to go to Rangoon in Birmah [Burma, now Myanmar], and stay there for a time. It was my intention to give an introductory address before the English-speaking people there, and thus obtain pecuniary assistance to leave for another place. From there we were thinking of going to Hongkong, and thence to Japan, and [then] . . . to America. This project will perhaps appear very wild to an outsider, but to us it was a necessity, for we could not retract our steps to [the] Bombay Presidency, nor was it very easy to travel in Bengal or Panjab, where the zenana, as I have already informed you, is rampant. But, thanks to Providence, he has been reinstated in his former post.

That the couple, feeling cornered and threatened, planned to leave India to escape the sphere of British power altogether and seek asylum in America must indeed have appeared 'very wild' not only to 'an outsider' but even to another Indian. Perhaps the American avenue was too tempting under the circumstances; and the initiative seems to have come from Anandibai. In any case, Calcutta was perceived as having brought nothing but trouble.

My husband never lost anything before but in Calcutta; he had never seen police courts before but in Calcutta; we had never had scandals in our neighbourhood but in Calcutta; we had never seen double-tongued men before but in Calcutta. I do not know how much evil and misery is still in store for us. I have been telling him to sever his connection with the Government and be independent, to avoid any further calamities that may befall us, but he is wavering. He thinks it very difficult to earn a livelihood, but I think otherwise. Whether he is more experienced and knows the world better, and therefore cannot do anything hastily, or whether the more a man is advanced in position, and the more he gets beyond what is actually necessary to sustain life, the more susceptible of imaginary difficulties he becomes, I cannot say, but in my opinion man must fear nothing but God. As God is [above] us and supplies our wants, I do not know why we should have a thought for the morrow. Man wants but little, and for that little, he bears a world of care, which I do not understand. Let me be here, or in any part of the globe, I will get my bread.

But to return to your letter. I admire you for your sound principles and sublime thoughts. Had there been no difficulties and no thorns in the way, man would have been in his primitive state and no progress made in civilisation and mental culture. Your letter is a sermon which we needed. Each line is full of meaning and world-wide knowledge. I do not know how many times I should thank you. The purity of your heart and dignity of your character are in my humble opinion worth imitation by the wisest. Indeed I am so thankful to God for having given me an opportunity to find a good instructor in you.

We have our food cooked by ourselves. We do not get these things ready-made in the Bazar. As we had no pots with us in which to cook food, we could not but remain without it, till we had our pots and furniture brought home. We never employ low caste people to do our household work, and as we were but two, in a place where servants and other things available were of no use to us, we could not but remain fasting. Imagine, you go to a place where there are no shops and you have plenty of money in your pocket; there is nobody to give you food, what will you do with your money? I have told you before that as the people of India are not given to travel, there are no hotels for us at each halting place. When we go on a [journey] from one place to another, we generally take with us articles of food prepared in milk and sugar, without a drop of water, for anything prepared in water is not carried and eaten on the road unless it is prepared and eaten then and there on the spot. So money is not always a useful article in India.

Despite these hardships caused by the strict rules of purity, Anandibai does not seem to question caste differences or Brahmin superiority sustained at so great, albeit occasional, a cost. She is far more open to a critique of Brahmin marriage-related customs, but not at the price of ritual superiority. Both gender and caste issues were the thrust of the reform movement in Maharashtra, but like many of the other Brahmins, she perhaps remained insulated from the latter. Nor does it seem to occur to her that her bold plans to travel to Burma, Hongkong, Japan, and on to America would entail unending fasts. Furthermore, the couple was dependent on access to caste-fellows, and the effects of a long-term deprivation in this regard does not seem to have occurred to her.

Her repeated inquiries about Mrs Carpenter's supernatural experiences at last elicited the startling information that Anandibai's late father had appeared before her and prompted her to write to Anandibai.

> I am glad to see that you have at last disclosed the secret. I tried once to get out the truth from you, but [you] did not yield. I am glad to hear that it was my loving father who impressed you to write to me. I have dreams about my departed friends, but never feel their presence near me when I am awake. I have dreamt many a time of my going to America and holding long conversations with you & other friends. What does it portend?
>
> I am exceedingly sorry to hear of the attempt to assassinate President Garfield. He is still alive and it is our earnest wish & prayer to God that he may be spared long.
>
> I have no boils now. I enclose a letter for dear Eighmie, and hope she will write me again. Her hand is after your fashion. We are going back to Park Street.

*

Stranded in a land perceived to be alien and even hostile, without family or friends, with her husband suspended from his job on suspicion of treason, Anandibai still had the strength of mind to devise solutions. To escape the stigma anywhere in British India they turned their thoughts increasingly towards America. Significantly, while Gopalrao understandably broke under pressure, she emerged the stronger of the two, and more resourceful and courageous. Her plan to give a public talk is the first sign of her stepping into the male-dominated public sphere which few Indian women had entered before.

Despite Gopalrao's being reinstated, Anandibai's negative attitude towards British rule and British officialdom remained strong. When she was eventually offered a job in the postal department, she turned it down without hesitation as a gesture of nationalist protest. The background for her decision came across in her letter to her brother-in-law, written from America in January 1886:

> There was a time when I had to humble myself before others for a job in the Post Office and was even offered a job suitable to my qualifications, at Rs 30 a month. But when time came to give a definite answer, I was loath to sell my freedom for this job or even for one offering me five times the salary. Now I have only one regret. My example could have helped many other women who are now struggling to get jobs.[4]

The domestic situation improved unexpectedly when the Joshees met the family of Raosaheb Dandekar, another Chitpavan Brahmin from Maharashtra.[5] Such was the strength of caste solidarity that the Dandekars immediately offered the Joshees a home away from home. It was from their address in Barabazar which Anandibai wrote on 17 October 1881:

On the 27*th* of August last we returned to Park Street and from the 30*th* I began to feel feverish till I was not able to cook. This necessitated my removal to Bara Bazar where a casteman of ours lives with his family. God is so kind to us that at the 11*th* hour, He showed me a house where parental care, kindness and affection are bestowed upon me. Had it not been for this, I do not know to what state of misery and distress we both would have been reduced. But thanks to Providence, the gentleman with whom I am living now immediately came to my assistance as soon as he heard of my illness. He insisted upon my being taken to his house. He came there at about 9 p.m. with an aged lady, thinking that my husband would not consent to send me at night; in that case the lady would remain with me [the] whole night and I might accompany her in the morning. What do you think? Is it not God Who inspired him to take care of me? This adds to my conviction which has taken a firm root in my mind that God will not forsake me, wherever I go either in India of abroad I will never lack kindness and care in His Kingdom. His wife treats me like a daughter.

Your letter is so interesting and full of motherly affection that I am sorry I was not able to thank you better. We are thinking of going out for [a] change, but don't know when we will. I will let you know of it when settled.

The pragmatic Mrs Carpenter seems to have suggested that Anandibai could solve the problem of looking conspicuously different by changing her dress. Frankly, this sounds no more feasible in India than it would have been in the United States.

Your advice to change dress is indeed reasonable, but to my mind very difficult to act upon. I remember having read in your letter that you found it very difficult to stick to your liking as to dress etc., and then gave way. It is so with me. My walking about in my dress is, [in] one way, productive of attraction to our people different in manners and customs, but if I put on a different dress, I will, I am afraid, expose myself to ridicule and contempt and laughter of those whose dress I have imitated. There are many natives who have adopted European dress for themselves and their wives, but are looked down upon by the gentry and the Europeans in general. A native in English dress looks like a butler. Besides I am reliably informed that even in America, people give respect to pure blood and not to mixed classes, such as Eurasians and half-castes. If I were to appear in America with [an] English dress on, I am informed, I shall not be admitted in high circles. Is it true, Aunt, that your people have such prejudices? When at Kolhapur, my husband had requested one Colonel there to our house for 'Pan Soopari' [a small social function with snacks], he did not come saying that he was a gentleman; so he and his wife would not go to those who were below their dignity; in England they had their rank; they were not like these missionaries who had no position at home. Man is full of vanity. To tell you the truth, there are many of his stamp in India. So you see how difficult it is to live in this world.

In view of the interminable discussions about Anandibai's dress, which were later to follow her entry into the limelight, her reasoning about not wishing to change her dress for fear of appearing undignified is revealing.
As a way out of their difficulties, Mrs Carpenter seems to have made an offer of financial help, perhaps to enable Anandibai to go to America.

I don't wish to put you to any expense on my account. I am confident that I shall make my way into any country without money in my pocket. All I wish from you is your never-ceasing kindness and good graces. I must first prepare myself [to be] worthy to visit your land. I have taken up Sanscrit [sic] to show to your people what precious treasure our Vedas and Shastras contain. I have made myself acquainted with all Puranas [and the epics].
It is, however, also encouraging that you will also extend a generous hand to me. I know God has sent you down on earth to do good to mankind, and I will be one of many millions who are blessed by you. My husband is exceedingly thankful to you that I have in you a true hearty and sympathetic well-wisher and joins me in wishing love and respects to self and husband. . . .
Before closing I beg to acknowledge receipt of your favour of 1st September last with two tins of herbs. I shall use them according to prescription. I hope they will do me good.

A month passed before Anandibai picked up her pen again on 14 November 1881:

> I have just returned here. I was so many days at Bara Bazar. I am now perfectly recovered. . . .
>
> This year from the 1*st* October till the 9*th* November I used to get up at three in the morning and go to the river Ganges for bathing and returned before dawn. I had two other female companions to accompany me. In Bengal respectable women go to bathe in the Ganges early in the morning that they may not be seen by men, but are exposed to attacks and outrage of modesty and sacrifice of chastity at the hands of ruffians and bad people. This period is considered auspicious and those who perform these early baths attain merit and their sins are consequently washed away. I shall not take up your time in dwelling upon the questions whether it is religiously meritorious or not, but it gives you a habit of early [rising] and exercise and keeps a man healthy.

Whether these early baths had any detrimental effect on Anandibai's already eroded health is not known.

> I am glad to tell you that we shall be leaving Calcutta very soon. My husband is posted to Barrackpoor, 14 miles from Calcutta. You will therefore direct your letters in future to the care of 'The Post Office, Barrackpoor, Bengal". I hope we shall be very comfortable there. The clouds will be lifting and brighter prospects dawning as you sincerely wish. Calcutta is the capital of India, where all high officers live, but it is to us an imprisonment. Here I could not make acquaintances and if I did I found it difficult to keep, as we live so far from one another.
>
> The death of the American President is a national loss deeply mourned by the Indians. There is not a single paper in India which has not devoted a column or two in mourning the loss and describing his noble character. Blessed must be the land in which such a bright star was born, blessed must be his mother.
>
> You have clearly set forth the responsibilities of parents towards their children. How few mothers in India understand them? How many children are daily driven to the verge of <u>absurdity</u> and ignorance for want of proper care and tuition on the part of their parents! It is indeed very useful to rear

children in righteousness and truthfulness, but how seldom are we successful. . . .

I do not know when I shall realise the reality of the spiritual world. India is becoming alive to the truths of spiritualism. There are some good mediums here in Calcutta through [whom] messages are received. . . .

Yours affectionately
Anandibai Joshee

Notes

1 Pandita Ramabai, *Stri Dharma Niti*, 3rd ed., Kedgaon: Pandita Ramabai Mukti Mission, 1967 (1882), p. 8. For a translation, see Meera Kosambi, *Pandita Ramabai through Her Own Words*, Delhi: Oxford University Press, 2000, pp. 35–101.
2 The term *zenana* is used loosely to indicate varying degrees of women's seclusion within the home.
3 Simla was the hot-weather station of high British officials.
4 Kanitkar, *Anandibai*, pp. 78–79.
5 Ibid, p. 69.

5

THE BENGAL INTERLUDE
Serampore

Anandibai's next letter went on 26 December 1881 from Barrackpore, a sizable British military cantonment town about eight miles north of Calcutta.

. . . I am much better now, at least free from fever. . . . I daily grow stronger in my faith in spiritual communications. (To tell you the truth, I always labour under inward impression. I solve many difficult things while sleeping. I was not able to cut different kinds of native dresses for men and women, but I have learnt them in dreams. . . . Next morning when awakened I actually did the same according to memory and found everything fit and complete. Whenever I have to learn anything by heart, I do it when asleep. In the day I read the passage to be committed to memory but once, and in sleep I read it over and over, and repeat it the [the] next morning without a mistake. Whenever I find any difficult passage in poetry I pass it over in the day, but in sleep I paraphrase it correctly and the next morning I am alright in translating it. I do not know who teaches me, but I make progress thus.) . . .

As I am not familiar with the English or American houses, I do not know how to satisfy your curiosity about the city house. But we were living in a house which was like those in which Europeans live in India. . . .

As you are not born and brought up in [the] Hindu religion you will not, I am afraid, appreciate its true merits. No religion is bad, but its followers and selfish interpreters [are]. Our priests are prejudiced and corrupt as are those of other religions. I dislike them as a class. I would rather be ignorant and illiterate than to have partial knowledge of everything. As you value sickness as a means for the enjoyment of happiness, so I regard irreligious people as pioneers of true knowledge of this world. Had there been no priesthood, this world would have advanced in civilisation ten thousand times better than it has now. So you need not expect to learn anything from our priests, who are no doubt groping in darkness. The spiritual truths which lighten all burdens and call for no sacrifices, are our moral teachers. Our forefathers used to commune with the all-pervading force and derive knowledge therefrom. They disregarded external duties and put too much stress on the acquirement [sic] of self-knowledge for the emancipation of the soul.

Then was the promised description of a Bengali wedding performed according to the Brahmo Samaj rites.

I am glad to inform you that if I have at all received any school-ing, it was for a year only, when we were in Bombay. It was a mission school [where I was compelled to read the Bible]. . . . on the whole though I have nothing to say against the Bible, which is a code of ethical rules, except the command, 'he that believeth shall be saved' and 'he who doth not shall be damned'. I have all along found the missionaries very head-strong and despising the faults of others. How arbitrary would it be if I were to say that all you believed was nonsense, and all I did was just and proper. My dear Aunt, I have nothing to despise. The whole universe is a lesson to me. I am required by duty to respect every creed and sect, and value its religion. I therefore read the Bible with as much interest as I do my own religious books.

I sincerely thank you for your undivided sympathies with me and my husband in the sudden fall into the depth of unsur-mountable [sic] anxiety and distress brought about by that sad event. If I had been called to share the storms with my husband, I would have done nothing but my duty which I owe him as his deserving wife. There would have been nothing commendable and heroic. Let there be any amount of difficulties and distress, and I think I shall be more than equal to face them.

Religion as a topic for discussion seems to have been broached for the first time. Anandibai's pride in Hinduism, coupled with a liberal acceptance of all religions, paralleled her combination of nationalism and appreciation of Western advances. Also consistent with her charac-ter were her impatience with religious intolerance, the falseness of the priesthood of all religions, and the Christian missionary propaganda – all of which were to be voiced again in her later letters.

*

The year 1882 dawned without ushering in any substantial change. Anandibai sent a postcard to Mrs Carpenter on 16 January 1882.

In April 1882 Gopalrao was transferred to Serampore, the former Danish trading town situated on the west bank of the Hooghly, across from Calcutta. The predictable, strict gender segregation denied her unrealistically optimistic expectation of female company, and the alien customs of Bengali women (such as habitual chewing of the betel leaf, which stained their mouths red) seemed improper to her puritanical tastes, especially because in Maharashtra usually only prostitutes followed this practice. She could obviously not free herself from this prejudice. Her first letter to Mrs Carpenter from Serampore on 18 April 1882 said

> as intimated in my last letter, we left Barrackpore on the first, and arrived here the same evening. The river is only a mile wide, and we crossed in boats. Serampore is an old town of historical note. The first missionary college in India was established here. It is still flourishing. There are many rich landholders whose houses are princely. But the inhabitants are barbarous and superstitious as they were hundreds of years ago. If the men are friendly, they will not allow their women to associate with their own sex, they are foreigners like me [?]. I can form no acquaintance with them, unless I become a missionary and force my way into the zenana. You must not suppose they would not like to see the world, and yet some of the Bengali women who have been educated follow very barbarous customs [like chewing the betel leaf]. . . .
>
> I rely on God and do not seek to know who are his individual messengers to me. Take any religion you like and you will find that its founder was a holy man. Go to his followers and you will find holy men the exception. I am glad to inform you that Miss Dobson's school has been closed owing to her obstinacy. Soon after I left, she required all her scholars to read the Bible, and the result was that her pupils, ninety in number, left her, and she went home never to return.[1]

This news must have brought a satisfying sense of vindication.

*

The Joshees' socio-cultural orbit possibly expanded through two incidents. The first was the sudden widowhood of Pandita Ramabai upon the death of Mr Medhavi, a Bengali non-Brahmin and Brahmo lawyer, on 4 February 1882. Their inter-caste marriage had alienated Medhavi's family, and Ramabai had no family or relatives left, but was alone with a baby daughter. The Joshees wanted to befriend this famous fellow Chitpavan Brahmin and offered her shelter – though she gratefully declined it.[2]

The second incident was the death of Vishnushastri Chiplunkar, a socially conservative and militant nationalist mentor of B. G. Tilak, in April 1882. The deeply affected Anandibai wrote a letter to the Tilakite paper *Kesari* in Pune, in the heavily Sanskritised Marathi favoured at the time.[3]

From Serampore the Joshees undertook a sightseeing trip of North India, from the holy city of Banaras, the former Nawab of Oudh's seat Lucknow, the Mughal capital Delhi, and the planned city of Jaipur in Rajasthan. Anandibai wrote to Mrs Carpenter:

> Our visit to Benares was not planned as a pilgrimage. Benares is a lovely place. On our way back, we spent only twelve hours there. So it was not possible to see anything. Therefore we wanted to spend about 8–15 days there, then proceed to Lucknow to see the Kesarbag and Alighat fort (the like of which is not to be seen in the whole of India. It has flat ground on top and contains large five-storied mansions), then spend about a month at Delhi to see the Jumma Masjid and fort, and Vrindavan, which are all beautiful places, and then to Jaipur. Jaipur is a very large city and is constructed in such a way that from one gate one can clearly see the opposite gate. This is true of all the eight gates. After seeing all these different places, we had planned to return to Benares and then back home again.

The letter of 16 May 1882 was also addressed from Serampore:

> Your favours of March and April are with me for reply. At the head of each letter are beautiful pictures which are really worth looking at. . . . .
>
> I am very much interested in the work you do from morning till evening. Your habits are really ladylike. You will find the women in this country both rich & poor employing their time as usefully as you do. . . . But alas! How few are [there] among [the] European residents in India, who act in the footsteps of their forefathers or ladies at home.

My time is not so usefully employed as yours, but I will give you an account of the life which the generality of our women lead. We get up at five o'clock. After answering the calls of Nature, which is the primary duty without which no person is clean to do any other business, much less to worship God and prepare food, we sweep the ground and wash all the copper and brass pots used for drinking purposes and worship, then oil and comb and dress our hair fixing several kinds of ornaments in them. Then if there be children in the house, rice is prepared for them at about half past seven. Children eat it with salt and ghee put into it. Ghee means melted butter. Milk is sometimes used with rice. Children use pickles [and other condiments]. We commence to give rice to children when they are one year old. Hand-made breads of wheat flour are sometimes made for children's breakfast. . . . As soon as vegetables are brought home from the market, we wash them first, and then cut them into small pieces. So are rice, pulse, and wheat flour cleaned and kept ready in dishes for cooking. We generally prepare five or six vegetables and an equal number of sour, hot and sweet arti-cles [like a form of salad]. . . . our stove is earthen by the side of which we sit, after bathing and changing our night clothes and putting on sacred ones which are dried in a room where nobody will go and touch them. First we put an iron pan or a brass pot on the stove and put [a] little oil in that. When it is hot, [mustard] seeds are thrown into it. So are cumin. When they are properly broken and fried, we put the vegetables in it. We take our meals twice a day. The first meal is at about twelve. And the second at seven to eight p.m. as a rule, men take their meals before females who serve.

Anandibai's detailed description of the daily meals, diet, cooking practices, and the state of ritual purity mandatory while cooking and eating is couched in a style easy for a foreigner to understand, and also conveys quite subtly the Indian woman's household drudgery, deference to men, and the extent of gender segregation within the home. This last, however, was mitigated in Anandibai's case because the family was just she and her husband, and they had a friendly relationship.

A married woman does not dine until she has served her hus-band. After dinner men go to bed, and we are engaged in removing and washing the dishes and plastering cowdung on the ground [floor].[4] After this, we change our clothes and sit down [to] prepare for [the] next day's cooking, such as cleaning rice, etc. we then cut and sew our clothes if there be any till half past five, and then go to temples and return home after six or seven when we are again engaged in preparing articles for supper. This occupies our time till nine when we prepare our beds and sleep. This is what women in India generally do. They have no letters to write or books to read. They do not receive or give [make] calls except among their own female relatives. They do not speak with men, even with their own husbands in the presence of somebody.

I hope Helena has commenced to attending school. I am sorry I have not been able to send her presents on account of her birthday which fell on 19*th* March.

It is getting warm here and much sickness prevails in . . . my husband has been unwell. He has applied for one year's furlough. If he gets it, we shall start for America. It was our intention to secure a passage for Japan and thence to America, but it is a circuitous route and expensive. So we will be going via England. Can you tell me how many days it takes from England to America and what is the fare? I suppose Roselle is not very far from New York.

I have much pleasure to inform you that I had some Bengali ladies invited to my house one evening and I was very much astonished to see them bow down before me as if I were God. They were peculiarly interested in my dress and ornaments. They said that [Maharashtrians] had a respectable dress of their own, while they were half-naked.[5] . . .

I enclose in this letter some Indian leaves and flowers. My love and kisses to you all.

Social interaction with Bengali women was a rarity which Anandibai had bemoaned and the small get-together obviously did much to alleviate her loneliness.

*

The Joshees' much-awaited trip to America kept on being postponed, though Gopalrao was so fired with this ambition as to apply for two years' leave of absence, which was refused.[6]

Anandibai regaled Mrs Carpenter with an account of the Hindu thread ceremony and the tale of Satyavan and Savitri in her next letter dated 17 June 1882.

I am sorry to inform you that our starting for America has been postponed for about six months, as a furlough cannot be had before. . . . I shall not be restored to a peaceful mind until I hear that you are recovered from your illness.[7]

The rarity of Mrs Carpenter's bouts of ill health seems to have sent Anandibai into a panic.

Anandibai's American dream was rekindled by a letter from Mrs Carpenter which was filled with practical information and advice. In an ecstatic response, Anandibai poured out her revised plans. Initially the couple was to go together, but now she was to go alone in view of the expense involved and Gopalrao's financial responsibilities for his family. Besides, by sending Anandibai alone, he could set an example of a Brahmin woman going abroad by herself.[8] Anandibai camouflaged her anguish at the proposed separation from her only emotional anchor in life with notions of 'duty' and her 'country's needs', as well as genuine excitement, as she wrote from Serampore on 12 August 1882:

. . . I imparted my joy to you in a few words. As I was reading [your letter] I was in ecstasy, when it fell from my hand. For a while I knew not what to do. I wished I had feathers [i.e. wings], to flit at once. On that day I did not eat my food as usual, for my head and heart were full with joy and I thanked the Almighty for the approaching pleasure.

You know at first our intention was that we should both start for America. I remember that you too, a year ago, expressed your wish that we both go, but now it is altered. After serious deliberations we perceive that it will be very expensive. You can imagine how difficult it is for a small purse to pay for two passengers from India to America. Besides, my husband has an old mother and younger brothers to care for. I have neither a jealous nature to be hurt by this separation nor anyone to care for except my husband. I have had here two dear things above all one of which I have lost (through her disapprobation), and that is my mother. The other is my husband. I have two sisters and a brother. Oh poor mortals! They are under a kinsman's care quite ignorant of this world. So I am untied [without ties]. I am therefore prepared to go alone to America, in company of any respectable family. My husband will be here. Considering the future prospects of my life as a physician I must make up my mind to be separated from my husband.

You have reason to think that [a] very distant voyage will be hazardous for a girl of eighteen because the world is full of frauds and dangers, but dear Aunt, wherever I cast my glance, I see nothing but a straight and smooth way.[9] I fear no miseries. I shrink not at the recollection of dangers, nor do I fear them. Wherever I will be, there will [be] Heaven for me. I am sure God has created many high souls, like you, who will not neglect me.

Besides, we are never sure that we shall live unseparated *forever*. We know not when we shall be condemned to separation. Is it not always possible that one of us will be lost? I give an instance for your satisfaction. . . . if this life is so transitory like a rose in bloom, why should one depend upon another?

Everyone must not ride on another's shoulders but walk on his own feet. Perhaps my husband will follow me some time after, but I must not wait for him, as time is so precious.

Thousands are too violently attached to the contrary opinions. Hundreds show their own scruples by urging that I am liable to go astray and lead an unchaste life when unprotected by any nearest relative. My design meets the approbation of a few, say one or two to a thousand, and they are probably youths, reformers and patriots. You will easily believe that I, fearing the disapprobation of the many, will desist from my determinate [determined?] proposal, but it is not so. Though I cannot teach courage, I must not learn cowardice, not at last leave undone what I so long since determined to do. I am not discouraged. I only wonder at their scruples and their timidity. I am not sorry for their unfavourable opinions. Their opposition strengthens me the more. I promise myself that if my efforts will be successful, I will rerun to my native country; otherwise I will not see India again. I must not fear but try my best and show all what we Indians are like. Our ancient Indian ladies were very wise, brave, courageous and benevolent, and endurance was their badge. Let it be my badge also. I am sure nothing will harm me, or if it does, it will be for my good. I know that whenever any misfortune has befallen me, it has been profitable for me. As we are all children of one father, none will attempt to deceive or betray me, wheresoever I may be. No one has power to disturb and harm, except He gives it. We have neither the power of devolving misfortunes upon ourselves, nor the power of avoiding them. These must come according to His will. I must launch my fortune like a ship on the ocean of life. To what shore shall it go, to a fertile bank or a barren beach? Or will it go to pieces? Let me try to do my duty, whether I be victor or victim. So I have determined, and will start some time in December or January next. Please be so kind as to be there at the time. I am sure you will not seek to deter me from my purpose.

I am impatient to see you and to begin to learn what my country needs. I feel that the movement of my mind is due to the counsels of my husband. What he has taught me, he has so impressed on me that it will never be effaced.[10]

The local reaction to Anandibai's plans was predictably one of stunned disbelief, in an age when a closely guarded and protected upper-caste woman was not even allowed to step out of the house without a proper escort. The principal objections were the threat to her safety and chastity, the ritual objection to crossing the seas and eating forbidden foods, and a fear of her converting to Christianity under persuasion or pressure. These themes were repeated with minor variations by all her critics. Perhaps the hardest blow to Anandibai at this stage was the breach between her and the kindly Dandekars, who had cared deeply for her as their own daughter; they tried their best to dissuade her personally and also through Mr Ketkar and through Anandibai's sister, who wrote to inform her that their brother was on his deathbed. Gopalrao guessed this to be a ruse and stopped her from rushing home to see him.[11]

But support was not altogether lacking. Gopalrao approached Colonel Olcott of the Theosophical Society (which he had joined in Mumbai) for information regarding medical education for women in the United States; Colonel Olcott insisted on making Anandibai a member also, and gave her a letter of introduction to an eminent judge in America.[12]

Outwardly unperturbed, Anandibai continued her preparations, and entreated Mrs Carpenter for help:

Please find a couple of rooms for me in the house of some gentleman. My only desire is that he should treat me like a daughter. I am suggesting this because you do not live in the town where the medical college is. In case there is such a college in Roselle and if your house is large enough, please arrange accommodation for me there. But why do I worry when you know all this? But I must take care about my meals. I will cook myself, so that the expense will also be reduced.[13]

As the plan kept on being postponed, the optimum wait-ing period was over. In a state of uncertainty and suspense, Anandibai wrote on 17 October 1882:

There is not much to write about my departure for America. I am ready, but the company is still to [be found]. As I wrote to you earlier, letters have been sent to all the four quarters, but we have not found a family going to America. Missionar-ies and English people advise me to go directly to New York; to delay in England will be very expensive; so I am thinking of coming straight. It has been decided to embark at Calcutta and disembark at New York harbour. All this waste of time fatigues me. When a thing loses its utility and novelty, it is not liked any more. Man likes new and useful things so much and derives such indescribable [sic] joy from them, that he is willing to brave difficulties in his attempts to get new happiness. So, I am waiting for the present situation to change and to get new hap-piness even from trials, trouble and labour. The major obstacles have now disappeared. Only a good escort is wanting.[14]

At this juncture a strong ray of hope was provided by an Ameri-can couple, the missionary Dr Thoburn and his wife, Anna. Dr Tho-burn even inserted a notice in the newspapers about an escort for Anandibai.[15] Anna Thoburn, a former student of the Woman's Medical College of Pennsylvania (henceforth WMCP) wrote to Dean Bodley on Anandibai's behalf in late November 1882, albeit rather condescend-ingly. She also claims to have fitted out Anandibai with dresses she had consented to wear.

She will be a real curiosity. No doubt the first Hindoo woman who has ever set foot on American soil. I trust my native land will deal kindly with her. . . . She is a bright little woman – speaks English fairly well – and writes it better than I do. . . . She will no doubt appear dull at first as she will find it difficult to understand – but I think she will get on well after a time. . . .

The very next day, 28 November 1882, a buoyant Anandibai wrote to Mrs Carpenter:

Everything is going on through Dr and Mrs Thoburn. The doc-tor is old and very noble. . . . I do not know how to repay their kindness. I can only thank Him who gives them to me. [The name of the college Mrs Thoburn graduated from] is the

Woman's College of Pennsylvania at Philadelphia. I would like to go to the same College. She has already written [to them], but I must wait to consult with you. . . . I shall go with two English ladies of her acquaintance who will start in February. I am sorry to say that the Mahratta family who were so kind to me in Calcutta are wholly changed since they know I am going. . . . Their opposition is due to tender hearts, fearful minds, and foolish superstition. . . . [Now] nobody can hinder me.

God has given me two precious things, my husband and my aunt; so I have every happiness. You can understand how painful six months' separation will be for a loving couple, let alone six years. But separation is difficult to endure even for a day! You will see how I have hardened my heart, when I tell you that I will be happy with you though I am separated from him. I have given all my care and anxieties to Him who is the only Soul. He who separates us will bring us together again.[16]

Anandibai also wrote to Mr Ketkar outlining her plans.[17]

By 1883, the Thoburns were also alienated; they advised her unexpectedly to join a medical class to be shortly opened in Calcutta under Dr Thoburn's supervision, and turned hostile at her refusal to change her plans. Anandibai's new plan was to leave in February, with Gopalrao to go as far as Madras or Aden and leave her with some trusted friend. On 16 January 1883 she wrote to Mrs Carpenter that whatever happens, *'I will see America, the dream of my life, and I will stand or fall as I deserve'*. The situation continued to be fluid, but hectic preparations were underway. Anandibai bought a supply of saris, traditional khan blouse pieces, bangles, and the red kunku powder for the dot on her forehead, enough to last her three years. As she had given up foreign goods after going to Calcutta, she made warm clothes out of Marwar blankets. She conveyed this nationalistic resolution to Mrs Carpenter. Things remained unchanged in February1883.

Notes

1 Dall, pp. 53–54.
2 Ibid, pp. vi–vii.
3 Kanitkar, p. 310.
4 Anandibai had explained the smearing of floors with cowdung in an earlier letter.
5 Bengali sari.
6 Kanitkar, p. 90.
7 Dall, pp. 62–68.
8 Kanitkar, p. 91.

9 Anandibai was only seventeen at this time, but according to the Indian way of reckoning, eighteen, because she was in her eighteenth year.

10 Dall, pp. 69–73.

11 Kanitkar, pp. 114–15.

12 Ibid, p. 96.

13 Ibid, p. 95.

14 Dall, p. 74; Kanitkar, p. 95.

15 Kanitkar, p. 96.

16 Dall, pp. 74–75; Kanitkar, p. 98.

17 Kanitkar, p. 112.

6

'WHY DO I GO TO AMERICA?'

So widespread was the public outcry over Anandibai's plan that the Joshees' dwelling above the post office in Serampore was virtually mobbed every day. As a conciliatory action, Gopalrao proposed to defend the scheme publicly. But Anandibai undertook the task herself in a public address, 'Why do I go to America?' on 24 February 1883 at the College Hall in Serampore before a large audience.[1]

She selected and answered six oft-asked questions. First, 'Why do I go to America?' To study medicine and provide much-needed medical care to women – Indian and foreign – who were naturally averse to exposing themselves to treatment from male doctors. But there were at least some Western women doctors. She stated, 'In my humble opinion there is a growing need for Hindu lady doctors in India, and I volunteer to qualify myself for one'. Second, 'Are there no means to study in India?' In the solitary college at Madras and the midwifery classes in the three Presidencies, the education to women was defective and insufficient. Also, the harassment to non-Christian and non-Brahmo women going to these was considerable. Again, '[T]he instructors who teach the classes are conservative and to some extent jealous. . . . That is the characteristic of the male sex. We must put up with this inconvenience until we have a class of educated ladies to relieve these men'.

This was indeed a bold statement of male jealousy which had been hitherto unvoiced in the discourse about women's education. It had been independently presaged by Pandita Ramabai in Pune in September 1882 when she gave her testimony before the Hunter Commission on Education.[2] She said: '[I]n ninety-nine cases out of a hundred, the educated men of this country are opposed to Female Education and the proper position of women. If they observe the slightest fault they . . . [magnify] it and try to ruin the character of a woman . . . (cited in Bodley: xiv). This ideological imbrication was hardly surprising, because it was the women achievers who experienced the reaction of the threatened male hegemons. Although the Hunter Commission was to decide questions of elementary education, Ramabai raised the issue of medical education for women, which Dr Hunter took up privately in England, with the resultant formation of the Dufferin scheme to supply medical aid to Indian women. Ramabai's argument was that '[t]he women of this country are much more reserved than in other countries, and most of them would rather die than speak of their ailments to a man.[3] The want of lady doctors is, therefore, the cause of hundreds of thousands of women dying premature deaths'.[4]

'Why do I go alone?' was Anandibai's third question. Here, Anandibai emphasised her husband's family responsibilities as an irrefutable argument, precluding choice. Fourth, 'Shall I be excommunicated when I return to India?' This was dealt with through the common sense argument that religious observances and social customs could be violated as easily within India as without, so that being away made no difference to a religious person. But she also reiterated a vow to remain a Hindu in letter and spirit – to be invariably echoed in all later reports of her activities. Fifth, 'What will I do if misfortune befall me?' She relied totally on God for protection. Finally, 'Why do what is not done by any of my sex?' Because every individual decides on his and/or her own duties.

As to the charge of regarding the adventurous and frightening nature of her solitary voyage, Anandibai offered a multilayered answer: In practical terms, it was a necessary risk in the laudable pursuit of knowledge. In philosophical terms, it was part of the human condition that calamity and death struck everybody without exception.

Through this masterly strategy Anandibai explained and defended her plans, covering the most pressing queries in a manner that reached out and touched a sympathetic chord in each segment of a diverse audience. Her appeal to the audience was two-fold: Along the axis of gender, it was directed to Indian and Western women united by a common and identifiable need; along the axis of nationalism, to Indian men and women on grounds of cultural distinctiveness which rendered foreign women doctors with 'different manners, customs and language' clearly inadequate. The earnestness of this appeal, stemming from her own constant and often acute need for medical attention for about eight years following an early and painful childbirth, was obviously strong enough to communicate itself to the audience, as was her resolve – amounting to a firm feminist commitment – to help her similarly situated sisters.

As part of her effective strategy, based on her general reading and diplomatic bent of mind, she sprinkled her speech with allusions which would appeal both to educated Indians and to Christians.

The availability of medical education for women was a desideratum felt by the more progressive social reformers, and Anandibai captured the essence of the problem in its multiple aspects. The first was the traditional division of male and female spheres of activity. A denial of education to women was a basic tenet of the patriarchal ideology, and formal schooling for women was opposed to the extent of subjecting the students to all possible harassment and expressions of contempt, even in a cosmopolitan metropolis like Mumbai. Here, Anandibai throws an interesting sidelight on the leeway enjoyed by Brahmo and converted Christian women who were beyond the pale of Hindu orthodoxy.

Even when women's entry into the field of healthcare professionals was considered, their role was restricted to midwifery, a task supposedly routine and uncomplicated (or unimportant) and traditionally allotted to women; while men appropriated the more advanced and complex knowledge of *Ayurveda* – medical knowledge derived from the ancient Hindu texts or accessed in the newly introduced Western medical colleges. Either way, full medical knowledge was a male preserve. It is both interesting and significant that while women's basic education was being promoted by the male social reformers and treated as matter of persuading the orthodox society to permit the change, the few articulate women identified women's professional and medical education as a desideratum as well.

Interestingly, at about the same time, Pandita Ramabai was planning her own voyage to England to study medicine and answering similar objections to her going on her own with a baby daughter.[5]

Anandibai's public statement received wider publicity than could have been imagined. Under the rubric 'A Mahratta lady's Address', the *Theosophist* (April 1883, Supplement, pp. 7–8) reported 'the welcome news of another Native Lady, besides Pandita Rama Bai, to follow in the steps of that great Sanskrit scholar and orator':

> Mrs Anandi Bai Joshi [sic] . . . is so high in intellectual development above her country-women as to appear publicly and deliver lectures for the benefit of her sex. Thus she is very likely to become one of the earliest pioneers in one of the grandest and most needed reforms in India, that of female education and the enfranchisement of woman; her present comparative slavery in the Zenana being a pure anomaly, something quite foreign to old Aryan usage and forcibly adopted with the conquest of India by the Mussulmans [sic]. . . . we reproduce her speech found in the Indian Mirror. . . . we are happy to say

that since the above was in type Mrs Anandi Bai has joined our 'Ladies' Theosophical Society' in Calcutta.

Other (socially conservative) papers, such as the *Hindoo Patriot* of Calcutta failed to note the event. Even the *Mahratta* of Pune in its very brief and not so accurate notice in the column 'What the World Says', clearly attempted to sensationalise the event, citing Anandibai's charge of male jealousy for women's medical education. The paper perhaps classes her together with Pandita Ramabai as a staunch feminist.

Anandibai herself made a characteristically modest mention of the event to Mrs Carpenter on 27 February 1883: Her lecture at the Serampore College attended by a large gathering of natives, and a few Europeans.[6] On 6 March 1883, she added:

> After hearing of my lecture, Mr H. E. M. James, Director of the General Post Office of India, wrote to my husband: 'I was very glad to hear that Mrs Joshee has made her debut, and has succeeded. Pray give her my congratulations. I wish her every success. In recognition of her courage and public spirit, permit me to offer the enclosed cheque for one hundred rupees which may be useful to her'.[7]

Other letters of congratulations poured in. Mrs Summers, wife of the officiating principal of Serampore College, wrote: 'I was sorry not to have been present at your lecture. . . . but my husband told me that it was a great success, so accept my congratulations'.[8] Even Mrs Thoburn, no longer the kind friend she used to be, wrote Anandibai a letter of congratulations.[9]

Now Anandibai's preparations for her travel were completed. On 3 April 1883, an excited and distracted Anandibai picked up her pen to write to Mrs Carpenter:

> I sit down to write what may be my last letter, in happy antici-pation of the fervently hoped for event. Until I return to and write to you again, this must be considered my last letter! I have already informed you in my last letter that the steamer leaves on the 7*th*. Everything is settled. I feel relieved now that there is nothing to do but embark. By God's grace, this too will come about. My head is so full of joy that it cannot contain any-thing else. I have come to Calcutta with my husband; we are with a young and kind Mahratta friend. I have just come from the Consul-General of the United States [Mr Hans Mattson]

who has given me two letters of introduction. The summer is indescribable. I shall go on board on the evening of the 6*th*, and we shall sail the next morning. . . . A lot of work remains to be done. So as usual, I will excuse myself. Aunt, rest assured that we will meet very soon. The time draws near in which we shall be in one country and one place. Every moment short-ens the time. I cannot write more. I cannot prolong this letter because of the noise and tumult around. I am in such a state that I can't think of a single word or construct a single sentence. My regards to your husband and love to the children.[10]

Little did the happy and excited hour indicate that this was to be the last letter Anandibai ever wrote from India.

Notes

1 Dall, pp. 82–91.
2 PR and Hunter Commission. Rachel L. Bodley, in the *"Introduction"* to *Pandita Ramabai's The High-Caste Hindu Woman*, Bombay: Maharashtra State Board for Literature and Culture, 1981 (1887), p. xiv.
3 This was a sweeping statement; Ramabai only sought to draw an Indian-Western binary.
4 *Times of India*. (Reference unlocated)
5 Pandita Ramabai, *Englandcha Pravas*. – – For a translation, see Meera Kosambi, *Pandita Ramabai: Life and Landmark Writings*, London & New York: South Asia Edition, Routledge, 2016, pp. 102–121.
6 Dall, p. 91.
7 Ibid, pp. 91–92.
8 Ibid, p. 92.
9 Ibid.
10 Kanitkar, pp. 117–18; Dall, p. 93.

Part II

A PASSAGE TO AMERICA

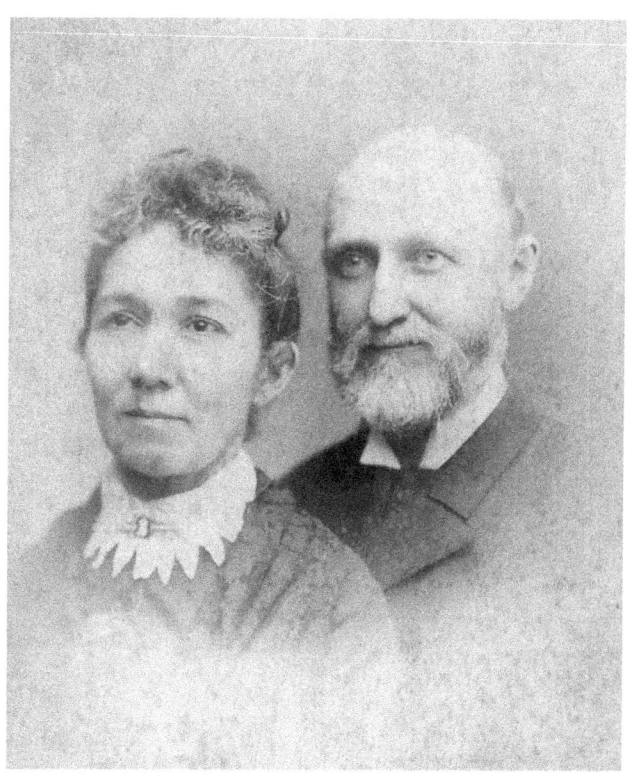

Figure PII.1 Mr and Mrs Carpenter
Source: Courtesy of courtesy William J. Cobb

7

CROSSING THE SEAS

My wife sailed yesterday morning by 'the City of Calcutta', in the company of many ladies who were strangers to her. She was to have sailed on Monday, the 9*th*; but early in the morning of Friday I received word that she must be ready to start on Saturday. We had invitations for the next three days, but could only decline them and hasten to get ready. She was not introduced to the ladies with whom she was to travel until she reached the ship, and even then her reception was cold indeed. Although at the eleventh hour, I advised my wife to expect nothing from them, but to trust Him who has made us both. My dear sir, I took good care of her until her departure, and now I hand over this precious charge to you and your worthy wife.[1]

With these words to Mr Carpenter, Gopalrao was able to report on 8 April 1883 that Anandibai was indeed on her way to America.

By now the event had assumed countrywide proportions and created a stir within Bengal as well as beyond. The *Theosophist* (May 1883, Supplement, pp. 6–7) continued to take a personal interest in her and report on her progress:

We hope that profiting from the grand privileges and facilities afforded to women in America, our brave sister may achieve there the greatest success. May she return from the Ocean of the Freedom an MD, having meanwhile avoided its two most prominent sand-banks: the Women's Rights Society and the Young Men's Christian Association, both of which classes, like the roaring lion in the desert seeking whom he may devour, are ever on the watch to entice at their arrival the innocent and the unsuspecting.

The paper cited an extract from the *Tribune* of Lahore which valorises Anandibai for her education and extraordinary moral courage. It hoped that her sacrifices and earnest patriotism would appeal strongly to 'the liberalism and conscientiousness of her fellow countrymen and society that may not be declared an outcast by them on her return. Backward Punjab, alas, has not got one single member of her sex who is capable of even sympathising with her object as, we believe, many of her Presidency will!' While wishing her every success, the paper hoped that other women – of any religion – would follow suit.

*

Anandibai's first communication with Gopalrao was a post card from London dated 10 May 1883:

> We disembarked safely at the Victoria Docks on the evening of the 9*th*. From there we walked a short distance to the train in which we travelled for about four miles. After walking another half a mile, we got into a hired carriage, and went to an inn as already arranged by the group. But it had no vacancies, so we came to this address [Lodging House] given above. The place is all right. Everyone has a separate bedroom and there is a common parlour. The weather is not very cold, but they say it is cold outside. I have not yet stepped outside. I might go today, but am afraid that people will laugh at my dress. I have a severe cold and also had fever yesterday. Today I am well. Don't worry. The fever must be due to the exhaustion of the voyage. The sky is clear. There is occasional sunshine. When we arrived yesterday, many said proudly, 'sometimes we get to see the sun!' later I will send an account of the houses and customs here. I cannot describe the terrible confusion about my luggage. Things like the writing box have gone to Liverpool. I have only the pen here, but the blotting paper, covers and writing paper have been sent ahead.
>
> We are all well. We will leave for America next Tuesday. I will send a detailed and really true account from America. Mrs Johnson is very good. Do not worry. Take care of yourself.[2]

A detailed account of the voyage was given, in view of its confidential nature, from the safe haven of Mrs Carpenter's house at Roselle on 25 June 1883. Gopalrao, already basking in the limelight, was quick to publicise it through the *Indian Mirror*, from which it was reproduced by the *Theosophist* (October 1883):

I received your letters from Puna [sic], Kalyan and Sholapur. My joy at seeing them may be better imagined than described. . . .

God has given me a strong, nay, hard heart which stood, and I hope will continue to stand, any trial or difficulty in the world. How many misfortunes must have befallen me in the space of 59 days, while travelling in remote foreign lands, I leave it to you to imagine. . . .

When I entered into the land of waters, I earnestly hoped that I would enjoy the sea without satiety, but I soon got weary of seeing what I saw once. I have had my repose disturbed a hundred times by the feeling of painful separation from home. Soon after I left Saugor, I felt sea-sick. Sometimes my companions pressed me to partake of meat, and when I refused to have it, they used to make fun of me in whispers. For almost a fortnight I had been a source of amusement to all. They did not take any interest in me. They thought no better of me than of a Native *ayah*! Once it so happened that I was seated on a sofa in the saloon when Mrs xxx came and told me to go and get on the deck, or any other seat I could find. I got up without saying a word, and went to the stewardess, for she called me in when she saw me going upstairs. 'It is very cold upstairs. You are not used to this climate. I am sure it will kill you. Do you like to go to the hospital in London where, I am quite sure, you will not like to stop a minute?' said she to me. 'Why don't you go and sit on the sofa? . . . You must be very careful', she added. To this I made no reply. [The] next day being Sunday, Mrs xxx asked me to go to the service. I said, 'I would rather sit with the *ayahs* than with those who think less of me than even the *ayahs*. . . .'

We left Calcutta on the 7*th*, as you know, and stopped in the midst of the river after a slow voyage of twenty-four hours. We again commenced sailing. I have already told you that we did not stop at Madras. On 12*th* April, I once heard that we were going to stop at Colombo, but I soon found that we were going further. We saw from a distance of about one and a half mile the rocks and mountains and hills of Ceylon. Now it was the close of the day. The sky was perfectly clear; the sea was serene; the sun had spread his beautiful garments over the lovely sea; the beautiful golden rays of the sun peeped into the dense coconut trees, which enhanced the beauty of Ceylon. Though I have not seen it myself, I venture to say that Ceylon must be a handsome place.

So happily we passed Ceylon, and arrived at Aden on the 20*th* of April at about 7 p.m. some of the passengers (both ladies and gentlemen) went ashore and came back before 10 p.m. it was the first time that I saw Africans. The physiognomy of the Negro is so peculiar that it is impossible not to recognise it at the first glance. His thick, protruding lips, his low forehead, his projecting teeth which peep out between his lips, his woolly and half-frizzled hair . . ., his beard, his short flat nose, his retreating chin, and his round eyes, give him a peculiar look amongst all other human races. The bones of the skull and those of the body are thicker and harder than those of the other races. Several are bow-legged; almost all have but little calves, half-bent knees, the body stooped forward and a tired gait.

Anandibai's description of the racial features of Africans above and of Arabs below sounds surprisingly technical for her understanding and vocabulary. One wonders whether Gopalrao had inserted the matter taken from some book and interpolated it in order to impress the readers.

On the same day we left Aden. On the 25*th* we arrived at Suez about 5 p.m. I saw another type of the human race. I mean the Egyptians. We did not go on shore, but I saw plenty of them on board the steamers with fruits, shells, necklets, bracelets, corals, large beads, photos, silk and golden clothes, pots, etc. The Egyptians are fair and well-made. The characteristic of the Arab race are a long face, a high forehead, a retreating, small mouth, even teeth, eyes not at all deep set in spite of the want of prominence of the brow, a graceful figure formed by the small volume of fatty matter and cellular tissue, and by the presence of powerful but not largely developed muscles, a keen wit and bright intelligence, and a deep and persevering mould of character [?]. You see, therefore that the Arab type is really an admirable one.

I am sorry I have forgotten to inform you of something about my food on board the ship. . . . You told me to write you all about my sorrow and joy. As to joy, I had none; nor did I expect any. . . . But as to my troubles, I had plenty of them, plenty for one like me. You might have thought that I was in abundance. Yes, . . . but not in what you would, perhaps, imagine. But let me thank God. . . . for His kindness in giving me strength to put up with all that befell me. . . . I had kept no connection with any lady (even with Mrs xxx). I had chosen an excellent companion that helped me to pass time quietly and pleasantly – I mean a book. I never felt lonely while reading. I read seven books on board the steamer . . .

Now in regard to my food, you might have thought that I could get whatever I liked. I could get a good many dishes, though I would not. Indeed I was well-nigh on the point of starvation. I was nearly starving for about seven weeks. What were dried fishes [sic] to me? What should I do with the soup they would serve me, and how could I sit among them, and see them swallow dish after dish? How could I stand the sight of long-long bones, etc.? How could I eat things composed of old vegetables, stalks, and half-rotten potatoes? It required a stronger stomach than mine to retain an appetite for such kinds of food. . . . My only food was two or three potatoes (for I could eat no more), I scarcely had rice, for it was too coarse and hard to be eaten. There were cakes that I liked most at first, but I grew weary of them, and to make my condition worse, my gum began to swell. It hurt me to eat, to speak, laugh, or to do anything else. Day by day the pain became more severe. It made my head ache. My stomach was still worse. This state of things lasted for nearly three weeks, when I thought I had better consult a doctor. A week elapsed before I found the doctor; for I could not catch his time. I saw him every day at table, but he went away before I left the table. So two days before our arrival in London, I consulted him. After hearing all particulars, he said that my wisdom teeth were just growing [and causing the trouble]. For three days I could not stand, nor sit, nor sleep. . . . my companions did not know of [any of this] till we were in London. . . . I have nothing to say against anyone. For they were all very kind to me after their own fashion. I had to suffer all kinds of inconveniences for the first four weeks or so. After that, they all became so fond of me that they were quite unwilling to part company with me. . . . so a few days before our arrival in New York, Mrs xxx said to me, 'Mrs Joshee, your husband has given you to my charge, and Mrs Carpenter cannot claim you from me; but you are married, and if you are not willing, I cannot keep you'. In New York when they bid me good-bye, they kissed me over and over again.

While reproducing this letter, the editors of the *Theosophist* prefaced it with their own extensive and indignant comment about 'our poor little voluntary exile' who turned a 'willing martyr'; her starvation on board the steamer, which should have taken better care of its passengers;

and the racial discrimination shown her by her Western 'companions'. This last was interestingly imbued with inverse snobbery and elitism on behalf of Anandibai's 'superior' Aryan roots.

The editors would have been even more outraged had they been privy to Anandibai's next communication on the subject to Gopalrao (of unknown date). This confidential account described the missionary ladies' efforts to co-opt her and wean her away from Mrs Carpenter, as well as interdenominational rivalries among the missionaries. Racial discrimination and forced starvation were also the lot of Pandita Ramabai, who travelled to England at the same time, in April to May of 1883. But she was accompanied by her two-year-old daughter and a female companion, and thus sheltered from the worst experiences that Anandibai had had.[3]

*

While Anandibai was progressing towards her destination, Gopalrao, back in India, was quite prostrate with grief and took three months' leave to travel. He wrote to her from Nashik on 15 April 1883, giving her a graphic description of his jumbled and uncontrollable emotions of grief and pride, and of the brusque manner he had assumed in an effort to hide them from her. Nowhere is the contrast between his excitable nature and Anandibai's usual calm and sober tone clearer. Gopalrao's travels brought him eventually to Madras, a visit reported in the *Theosophist* (June 1883, Supplement: p. 12) in view of his newfound celebrity.

If Gopalrao's friends and acquaintances in Bengal and Maharashtra were largely hostile to Anandibai's travel abroad, so were Anandibai's parental family. They vented their criticism, not unmixed with curiosity, through a (Marathi) letter which her younger brother Vinayak was made to write from the New English School, Pune, in July 1883. After asking her whether she went voluntarily or was forced by Gopalrao, whether she took along her jewellery, about the climate and food in America, and other quite irrelevant and ignorant questions, he ended with an English flourish issuing a dire accusation: 'Mrs Anandibai Joshi! You have done no right, because India is your native place'.[4]

Notes

1 Dall, pp. 93–94.
2 Kanitkar, pp. 145–46.
3 Ramabai, *Englandcha Pravas.*
4 Kanitkar, p. 133.

8

CULTURAL ENCOUNTERS

Weary of limb and depressed in spirits, Anandibai reached the United States on the 4th of June, to tumble into the welcoming arms of Mrs Carpenter at New York Harbor. The sense of the historic and the dramatic was underplayed as usual in her matter-of-fact report to Gopalrao:

> On the 16*th* I left London for Liverpool and sailed for America the following day at 3 p.m. by the S.S. City of Berlin. We reached Queen's Town on the 18*th* at roughly 10 a.m. We were to go further the same day, but the engine got into disorder. We were, therefore detained there for more than a week. We arrived in America on the 4*th* . . . at noon. Mrs Carpenter came aboard the steamer to receive me.[1]

After reaching the Carpenter residence, her home away from home for the next few years, Anandibai gave way to a welter of emotions – relief from prolonged tension, homesickness, and the daunting prospect of a demanding course of studies – which even she was forced to acknowledge:

> When I saw all the letters waiting for me, I instantly burst into tears. My heart was heavy and my eye swollen. I passed a few minutes in this state when I at once started. I blushed at the display of my own weakness at a time and place like this. I blamed myself. . . . I got up and took the letters, and stepped down to where Mrs Carpenter was sitting. It was now five o'clock. I was rather tired. My head was warm. The day was hot. Then I wrote my letters to you.[2]

Before Anandibai had had time to grasp the full contours of her new world, friends and neighbours rushed in to greet the newcomer with warmth and affection not untinged with curiosity.

> Visitors began to pour in. . . . So, in the space of a few hours, [many] visitors called. It was past ten and they were coming. At last Mrs Carpenter was obliged to shut the windows so that no one could see me [inside]; and so I escaped them. It was a happy day. They called it a holiday. They said the sun was so bright that day that they never saw anything like it. I was seated in a rocking chair with flowers in my hands. Lady friends came, embraced, and kissed me, and gave me flowers. Since I left you I have had nothing but kindness. . . . We have hot weather, green grass, loving trees, pleasant breeze and flowers, cool wind, kind friends, and comfortable rooms. Helena is a sweet little girl, and Eighmie a clever, studious companion. I am so happy. Do not be discouraged. Remember the good old maxim, 'Let patience have her perfect work'.[3]

There was a general expectation that Anandibai would be excited and confused by her encounter with this vastly different society and culture. In fact, before leaving India, she had warned Mrs Carpenter about her limited exposure to Western society: 'As I do not visit Europeans very frequently, I am ignorant about your manners. You might think me vulgar or uncivilised. Also, the difference in our customs might compel me to ask frequent questions which you might find tedious'.[4] Mrs Carpenter had already resigned herself inwardly to this prospect, only to be surprised and impressed by the eighteen-year-old girl's calm and controlled reaction, as she confessed later:

> Anandibai talked neither more nor less than necessary. Such dignified behaviour is rare even in a much older person, whether American, Hindu, or native of any other country. . . . [When we first boarded the train together in New York] I expected that, like other immature young girls, she would also push her head out of the train window and stare at things she had not seen before, or ask me about them. But no such thing happened; she just sat quietly. On several occasions I thought she would be curious. I volunteered information but she herself asked no questions. This was an indication not of mental sloth but of quiet observation. As I found out from her later remarks, she had observed keenly and with a sense of discovery whatever

passed before her eyes. She never asked tedious questions about the novel sights and customs, and never bothered about her surroundings. Her conduct was irreproachable. Anandibai's every act was done with skill and concentration. Her neatness and tidiness are qualities which others may do well to emulate.[5]

The curiosity about Anandibai was natural because her reputation preceded her. It was almost as a celebrity that she stepped onto American soil. An article accompanied by her photo (see Plate 2) had already appeared in *Frank Leslie's Illustrated Newspaper* (12 March 1883) under the rubric 'Mrs Anandibai Joshee: Leader of the Movement for Woman's Emancipation in India':

> We give on this page a portrait of Mrs Anandibai Joshee, a Brahmin lady of high social standing, who has recently produced a sensation in India by breaking away from the fetters of Hindu thought and customs, . . . It is, of course, known to all that the position of woman in India is one of miserable degradation. . . . but no such pronounced action has been taken by anyone as by Mrs Joshee.

The paper also stressed Anandibai's heroism and courage in crossing seas.

> A warm welcome was also extended to her by the Methodist Church, with its tradition of sending women doctors to India, in an article by Mrs J.T. Gracy published in Spring 1883.[6] After tracing her background and courage, the author ended: 'We bespeak for her here, in this Christian land, sympathy and affection of all women who have at heart the upliftment of woman in all countries'.

*

Anandibai was sustained by her lifeline to India and to Gopalrao during the early homesick days, as she wrote on 27 August:

> I cannot describe the joy I feel on receiving your news so frequently. It is the only avenue for contact with you, for which I shall always be grateful to God. . . . Day and night I think of writing to you, and you never leave my heart! Even when my hands are busy, my mind is concentrated on just one subject. Only when I study is it directed towards my lessons, not willingly, but by force. . . . When I think of you, I am infused

with enthusiasm and hope. But sometimes the thought of you being in one part of the world and I in another, brings such disappointment that it shows on my face, and I feel afraid that people might notice it. I try my level best to suppress the disappointment, but how long can one succeed? In the beginning I often stifled the desire to weep. I have vowed never to let anybody see my tears. But now-a-days, I don't even feel like crying. My eyes are quite dry! Sometimes also the tongue seems dry and the throat constricted as if I am suffocating! I think the very tears have vanished from my eye or dried up! When the throat becomes full, there is but one way of clearing it – heaving loud sighs. But one needs privacy for that. It is bad manners to sigh in front of others. What a problem![7]

Probably in the same letter she continued – and this extract was reproduced in *Kesari* (6 November 1883), obviously as part of Gopalrao's publicity campaign:

My copies of 'The Mahratta' and 'Kesari' arrive regularly from Poona. The 'Indian Mirror', 'Subodha Patrika' and 'Natyakatharnava' also arrive on time; the 'Native Opinion' has not started yet. The nose-ring and pearls from Bhaskar have arrived. The nose-ring is all right, I adjusted it. The pearls in the gold chain are small. In truth, I did not need either of them. I have with me whatever I need. I have maintained my dress and diet pure, that is, in the traditional Indian style. I live in the midst of meat-eating people in their own country, but I am exactly as I have always been. Do not lose courage because of what people say. God cares about me. He will guide my judgement. Not only do I not eat their food, but on the contrary, I make them eat mine. Sometimes I cook for them, and they really enjoy it. Aunt even says, 'We are becoming Hindu day by day'. One day, Aunt, Eighmie, Helena, Mrs Deaden, her daughter and a couple of other [women] wore saris and 'kunku', and became totally Hindu!! At home it is a great fashion to wear saris. Even dolls demand saris! I have changed everybody's name and given them Marathi names with the same meaning, like Tara for Helena, Saguna for Mrs Stuart, Premala for Eighmie, etc. I address Aunt as 'Mavshi' [Marathi for Aunt]. In the morning everybody says 'Namaskar' instead of 'good morning'. Such is the state of affairs here.

Anandibai's determination to make the cultural encounter emphatically mutual was sure to please every Indian, especially Maharashtrian. Gopalrao was quick to assess the popular appeal of the letter and had it published in *Kesari* along with the following description of Anandibai's banquet for the Carpenter family and their friends at the beginning of September:

> Last week I attended an American banquet and gave an Indian one myself. Altogether eighteen places were set. There were all the proper arrangements including wooden seats and *rangoli* designs.[8] The sitting arrangement was on the floor, and flowers and perfume were distributed. The company was utterly delighted at the arrangements. The special dishes were as follows: rice, lentils and lemon, five vegetables, five salads, *puran poli* and sugared rice, *ladoos, vadis, karanjis, chirotas*, sweet mango preserve, and mashed banana with sweetened milk.[9] All the women wore saris.[10]

Mrs Dall gives a more detailed description of this feast, presumably based on Mrs Carpenter's own account:

> She was never weary of talking about her dear native land, and this summer she gave a great treat to her Roselle friends by improvising for their benefit a Hindu feast. Mrs Carpenter was living at this time in a large house. All the furniture was removed from the dining-room, and the smooth inlaid floor was ornamented and divided by delicate strips of red and white about four inches wide [to make one square for each guest]. Including Anandibai there were eighteen guests. . . . [T]he powder had been brought from India. . . . [F]resh green leaves of the buttonwood had been sewn together to do service as plates, instead of the long banana leaf which would have been used in India.[11] . . . Smooth pieces of board were placed . . . within each square to take the place of chairs. Small plates were set near the leaves in the corner to hold rice and curry. Sweetmeats were also served in small dishes. . . .
>
> The ladies were all dressed by Anandabai [sic] in bright-bordered Indian sarees which she took from her own wardrobe. . . . A Sanscrit [sic] prayer was reverently offered, and then the dishes . . . followed by coffee. As soon as each guest was supplied . . . Anandibai entered the square reserved for her, and prepared to teach her guests how to eat like a Hindu.

None of them dared begin until she had taken her seat. Anandabai would pick up a morsel, bring it a few inches from her plate, and then with a dexterous twist of her fingers toss it into her mouth. It seemed to fly magically to the right spot. 'To miss', she said, 'would be vulgar.'[12] After dinner, the guests repaired to the parlour, where a large mat had been spread, and huge white cushions had been provided for the ladies to lean upon. Every married lady had the scarlet mark on her forehead, and such bangles, necklaces, and other ornaments as Anandibai had been able to procure. To the ladies half-reclining on the mat, and to the gentlemen standing or squatting Hindu fashion on the floor, Anandibai distributed bouquets of flowers, and on the back of each right hand she left with her dainty finger a trace of attar of roses, which she took from a phial of green and gold.

The company was then sprinkled with rose water from a silver vessel, and Anandabai sat down, evidently considering that her work was done. Not so her guests – they had heard that Oriental dinners were wont to conclude with song, and at their earnest entreaty one tender ditty or one birdlike caprice followed another, until all were tired. It was a little singular that on this occasion all the guests seemed to approve of the unwonted cookery.[13]

*

Anandibai had left India, behind but India continued to tug at her through Gopalrao's often tactless letters and his desire to unburden himself. She continued to offer consolation and advice through letters, as she must have routinely done in person earlier:

> How can I tell you how sad I feel because of all the news you write to me! The sarcastic comments of xxx, the tantrum thrown by Raosaheb xxx, the mean behaviour of xxx while serving food, the marvel which you showed xxx, the shameful treatment of women during the chariot procession, . . . the contemptible rumour started by the people of Calcutta about you – I read all this with feelings of joy, sorrow, pity, overpowering sadness and heart-ache. . . . Never mind, there is no need to worry. You will not become what they say you are. I am saying this to console you, but don't think that my heart is not torn asunder. Honour is more precious than life itself. Even if I had a thousand lives, I would not hesitate to sacrifice them for my reputation. Even so, one has to face each day calmly. It is our duty to lead a pure life in the fear of God, no matter what people say and do. It is not in our power to shut their mouths,

and even if it were, one should not attempt it. They will shut up by themselves.[14]

About this time Gopalrao got himself into trouble through a quarrel with the postal authorities, and the following reference is possibly to his highest superior, Mr James.

> What you wrote about xxx in your last letter terrifies me. God forbid that such an eventuality ever befall you. If it does, remember that it will incur the grave sin of ingratitude. I am not trying to advise you; I don't have that right. But I am wrong. I do have the right to give you advice if I see that you are about to make a mistake. If I don't, I will fail in my duty and be an accomplice in your offence. You are greatly in xxx's debt. There is no hope of your repaying it, but the opposite might happen. Whatever happens, you have eaten his food, and I am convinced that you will not trouble him in any way. Do not hurt him by petty words or actions. He is old and hot-tempered. You are reasonable and compassionate. You revere him greatly.[15]

Elsewhere, Anandibai alludes obliquely to this trouble in a letter to her brother-in-law: 'You know as well as I do that it was my duty to apologise to Mr James for whatever my husband did. He knew whether he was doing right or wrong. . . . Mr James proved his true and sincere friendship. Now, whether Mr Joshee behaved accordingly? or not is another question.'[16]

Anandibai's primary preoccupation at this time was to arrange for Gopalrao to come to the United States, and she at once started making inquiries and plans:

> Whenever you come here, bring a good supply of clothes. Bring also several pairs of Chinese hand-made shoes, and things like stockings [western-style] coats, angarkhas [Indian-style cotton coats], warm and ordinary uparrnas [stoles for men], dhotars, pants, shirts, gloves, a good earthen water container (at Aunt's suggestion), etc. there are no earthen water containers here. Bring also a pair of sacred threads and a fine angarkha from Poona, without fail. Here the smallest thing costs a great deal and is not necessarily better than ours. Bring as large a supply of clothes as possible. In England I bought things like an umbrella, bag, blanket, gloves, etc. the same things cost four times as much here.

Mrs Jonson bought these things for me, saying, 'these things are essential for you. I am purchasing them here because they are very expensive in America.' Enough of that.

Aunt's husband wants you to bring along some Indian goods. In my opinion, you should bring tea. The people here are quite addicted to Chinese tea. So far they used to buy tea, which was thought to be Chinese, but was not. Some days ago, a gentleman here received tea from his brother in India and gave it to me. Since then all those have tasted it have enjoyed it a great deal. They look for it in the market, but do not find it. Even the gentlemen who never touched tea before toss off four cups at a time. In my opinion, it is essential for America and India to have trading arrangements. If this happens, our country will benefit greatly. A new law was passed last year to prohibit Chinese people (even women and children) from even disembarking in New York State, as you must have heard.[17] This means that no fake Chinese tea will be imported any more. Only the Indian source remains. If the tea is really pure, these people will jump at it even if it is expensive. Starting with tea, one can later explore what other goods will be in special demand here. It is true that the customs duty here is steep, even so it is my firm belief that a profit can be made after deducting the original price and the duty. I am quite convinced that honest trade will flourish here. With honesty in business and a well-founded plan, victory and wealth will be ours. What an excellent thing it will be if things work out accordingly. The traders in Poona are improving quite a lot these days. So, if possible, the hitherto non-existent connection between America and India should be established, and you yourself should take up this work and come here in the capacity of an importing and exporting agent. There does not seem to be any objection to this from your side. So let me know if the necessary arrangements can be made there, so that they can also be made at this end. If you are able to handle this, it seems likely that even Aunt's husband will make the arrangements here. He is also very keen that America should have some connection with India. So please do this, and inform me immediately. In the meanwhile my studies will also be smoothly under way.[18]

Anandibai's shrewd business sense certainly comes as a surprise, but seems to have been accepted without a question by her acquaintances in India. In fact the *Mahratta* (6 July 1884) was later to make a proud mention of her suggestion regarding the export of Indian tea to the United

States, in connection with its publication of extracts from the report of the Executive Commissioner for India at the Amsterdam Exhibition of 1883, emphasising that Indians were not yet aware of the great demand for Indian articles in Europe: 'our friend Mrs Anandibai Joshi' had also pointed this out. Thus, Anandibai came to serve as an unlikely conduit for information regarding business opportunities for India and Indians, simultaneously serving the nationalist agenda of withdrawing from the British yoke and seeking new Western pastures in America.

*

Similar other practical matters were discussed in the first letters which Anandibai wrote to Gopalrao. Probably in July or August, she wrote

> you have written that a student [from India] is planning to come here and that his expenses are estimated as Rs 250 per month. I laughed when I read this. This exorbitant estimate surprises me greatly. Although it is true that things are very dear here, it is extraordinary to spend so much to live like a student. If one wants to live in the style of a fashionable gentleman, then even this amount would not be enough! If I had such pretensions, I would never even have crossed the threshold, as you well know. How can our country afford to supply such a monthly amount? It would suffice to educate two students, and that would give twice as much benefit. But anyone who provides such information would be regarded as either foolish or ignorant. So you need not worry about me. I want to stand on my own feet and serve others. Let us pull on as far as possible, there are two of us. I have already come here, but you are also penniless. So if the fellow countrymen of this weak woman, alone in a foreign country, really take pity on her, they will help you in every way possible and send you here. And if that happens, it will be very convenient, as suggested earlier. It will serve their purpose as well as ours. Communication will develop between the two countries, trade will open up, and their purpose will be served without much burden. Only one question remains. When will this happen? . . .
>
> Your letter of June 12*th* arrived yesterday. Last week I did not receive a letter, so I suffered a great deal of anxiety. But then your letter arrived and I was relieved. My health is all right. Do not be anxious. . . . please send me your photograph, as I have requested you in my last letter. The money you send should not exceed 50 rupees, including transmission charges. The balance

should be put aside, so that it can be used for your passage. Aunt and her husband have asked me to convey their regards. They have also sent a message which I will quote exactly. She says, 'Your loss is our gain, and we are grateful to God for this. We are very happy in Anandibai's company', etc.

Aunt likes to tease a lot. The Andrus family is very nice. How wonderful it would be if I could draw an exact picture of how each and every person loves me! . . . I have no desire at all to hear xxx's praise. I would thank him not to do so. Real well-wishers never flatter. Never mind that. My eyes are eager for the sight of you. . . .

I beg you to accept the regards sent by everyone at home. I am returning some postage stamps which came here by mistake.[19]

*

At the beginning of September Anandibai started her private preparations for college.

Now only a month is left before I start college. Once the classes begin, there would be nothing but books and the pen, and no time either. Therefore I have made myself long-sleeved blouses out of the 'khun' blouse-pieces I had brought along. You had sent so many cloth samples from Madras, that I made a lovely quilt out of them. It is very beautiful as well as useful. I do not have enough saris for nightwear, nor are they necessary. So I have made three night-dresses out of plain white cloth. I have stitched six 'choli' blouses. Even when I go to college, I will do my own cooking and might spoil the saris. To prevent that, I have stitched six aprons which will also be useful in the surgery classes in College. I have sewn all these myself on the sewing machine at home. My sewing was so good that Aunt gave me the first rank!

I have learnt many new things. I help Aunt with the housework, and have earned a diploma in that subject, too. There are also Indian and local newspapers to read and letters to write. In my attempt to manage all this, sometimes I miss out on letters to you. What shall I do? It can't be helped, but I hope you will forgive me.[20]

On 10 September, Anandibai wrote to Gopalrao:

Your letter has arrived. My happiness known no bounds. Last week I was so restless because your letter had not come. That

114

is a thing of the past now. I am very uneasy to hear about your dream. I also had an identical dream on the same day! I don't know the meaning of this. My health is fine. All are well. . . . 'Native Opinion' and 'Indu-Prakash' arrived from Bombay in the last mail.[21]

In the midst of her acculturation process, Anandibai was being sought out by fellow Maharashtrians who had arrived in the United States earlier and regarded themselves as experienced advisers. Among them was one Mr Rajwade, whose Westernised manners quite antagonised her, as she confided in Gopalrao on 10 September 1883:

Bhaskar Vinayak Rajwade has come here. His seems to be a case of little action and much talk. His dress was quite English (even collar and tie!) and I quite disliked his hat. As soon as he arrived, he said he wanted to test me. I made no reply. I was waiting for him to repeat that, then I would have replied, 'The time for my examination has not come yet; when it does, I will invite you'. . . . Rajwade said, 'I have been to the theatre and am going again today. Will you come with me?' What impertinence! It is unbecoming for a gentleman to propose such a thing, and that too, to a decent woman. I told Aunt. I had already refused him. The man seems quite strange.[22]

Another Maharashtrian (identified in another letter as Mr Guruji) disgusted her by his crude behaviour, as she complained to Gopalrao:

When a man becomes thoughtless, there is no knowing what he may say and to whom. Matters are worse in the case of vulgar people; they have no idea how to treat decent people. And even if they do, they think of every woman as stupid and low. If they receive publicity in newspapers, they imagine that they have reached the highest peak of wisdom! They expect others to nod in agreement with anything they say! No matter how a man behaves in his own country, he ought to give up his contemptible ways and behave decently as long as he wants to stay in a foreign country. Probably only one or two persons leave India to travel abroad every year, but their good or bad conduct becomes a test case for the whole country. . . . if not for the sake of one's parents, one should improve one's conduct at least for the sake of one's country. But if a man disregards both country and parents, he may do what he likes. He has total freedom. But he should keep his own concerns and not attempt to destroy others' reputation. He owes it to his country. The man at the glass factory seems to have forgotten all this. To think that, like himself, others also travel abroad for the sake of self-indulgence and luxury is sheer narrow-mindedness![23]

*

The Carpenters had promptly made Anandibai answer a personality quiz (with thirty-seven questions), then in vogue; this 'mental photo-graph' dated 3 September 1883 and was recorded in Mrs Carpenter's album. After some questions about one's favourite colour, flower, tree, etc., come some serious ones. Anandibai answered that her favourite character in history was Richard the Lionheart; book to take up for an hour 'the Bhagawat Gita'; book to cherish (other than the Bible) 'the history of the world'; her preferred place to live 'Roselle now and here-after in Heaven'; her favourite characteristic, 'sincerity'; most detest-able characteristic, 'dishonesty and infidelity'; her idea of happiness, 'faith in God'; her 'bete noir', 'slavery and dependence'; the sublimest passion, 'love', her aim, 'to be useful', and her motto, 'the Lord will provide'.

While reproducing it, Dall stresses Anandibai's humility, sense of duty to others, faith, and religiosity.[24] Equally interesting is Anandibai's socio-cultural milieu, especially the dual cultural influences which moulded an English-educated Maharashtrian of the time. Taken together, the answers span Sanskrit works, Marathi devotional poetry, contemporary Marathi prose, and popular English authors. Her preference for the mango, jasmine, and the rose evoke the tastes and fragrances of India, just as the mountains bring memories of the majestic Western Ghats, which had watched over her early years.

Another personality exploration was an analysis of Anandibai's hand-writing, originally done in January 1881, which now received publicity through the *Psychometric Circular*, and which was promptly reproduced by the *Mahratta* in its editorial:

This is an intelligent, well-balanced mind, and cultivated with great care. It seems a lady with more than ordinary brain power, very independent, but not egotistical or intolerant. This mind seems directed to mental pursuits and the acquirement of useful knowledge; not afraid to investigate all or any subject, however unpopular. She is analytical and frank in speaking her mind. There is suavity of manner; she converses fluently and meets strangers with a cordial, graceful ease that wins confidence and esteem. . . . She has great equanimity of disposition, makes friends and is very appreciative of the attentions of refined people. . . . there is also great delicacy of character, womanly in every respect, very ardent in the love of nature, clings to old friends and associations, strong in the family ties. Her resolves spring from a holy desire to discharge her duty, regardless of self-sacrifice. She has a religious cast of mind, very conscientious and spiritual; . . . She has a fine memory; in [while] travelling nothing would escape her notice; has good descriptive powers . . . For the principles of truth, justice and correct deportment this lady has no superior. . . . She does not believe in oppression and will always defend the weak. . . . She has large hope which gives brightness to her life and an assurance that sustains her in this life of conflicts, and will not leave her until she reaches the shore of immortality. . . .

Very truly her friend,
Mrs C.H. Decker.
New York, Jan. 20, 1881.

Those who read the above and have the honour of the lady's acquaintance testify to the correctness of the above description.

While reporting this, the *Mahratta* seized the opportunity to present Anandibai as a model of Hindu womanhood, and stressed the contrast between her and Pandita Ramabai, whose recent conversion to Christianity in England had sent shockwaves of disapproval through Maharashtrian society.

As a relief from the above painful reading [of Ramabai's conversion] we take from an American paper called Miller's Psychometric Circular an extract. . . . We hope to give now and then this remarkable lady's [i.e. Anandibai's] progress at Philadelphia where she seems to have made up her mind to stay.

The *Mahratta* had begun to take serious note of Anandibai as a perfect foil to Ramabai, and continued to do so as long as Anandibai lived. Through her activities, which Gopalrao conveyed to newspapers, he ensured himself of considerable publicity in *Kesari* and the *Mahratta* of Pune, the *Theosophist* of Calcutta and Madras, and even American papers. The 'Pygmalion' had begun to make his mark in the world.

Notes

1 *Theosophist*, August 1883, Supplement, p. 6.
2 Ibid.
3 Ibid.
4 Kanitkar, p. 148, my translation.
5 Ibid.
6 The exact source is not known. The article was available in the Archives of the Medical College of Pennsylvania in January 1996.
7 Kanitkar, p. 156, my translation.
8 The small cylindrical device made of brass, perforated with holes, to make long strips of *rangoli* design is among the artefacts preserved by the family of Mr William Cobb, Mrs Carpenter's great grandson. It reminded me at once of this banquet description.
9 Puran polis are chapatis stuffed with cooked and sweetened chick pea flour, ladoos are sweet balls made with any of a number of flours, karanjis are half-moon-shaped fried sweets of wheat covering and a sweet stuffing possibly of grated coconut, chirotas are fluffy layered squares sprinkled with sugar or syrup, vadis are thick flat squares, made of some flour and sweetened. These are traditional Maharashtrian sweets.
10 *Kesari*, 6 November 1883, my translation.
11 Sometimes round plates made by sewing together large jackfruit leaves are also used in India. Bowls are also made of the same leaves.
12 This is surprising; the Maharashtrian custom is to convey the morsel directly to the mouth.
13 Dall, pp. 97–100.
14 Kanitkar, p. 129.
15 Ibid, pp. 129–30.
16 Ibid, p. 81.
17 The Chinese Exclusion Act of 1882.
18 Kanitkar, pp. 229–30.
19 Ibid, p. 232.
20 *Kesari*, 6 November 1883.
21 Ibid.
22 Kanitkar, p. 160.
23 Ibid, pp. 158–59.
24 Dall, p. xi.

9

ENTRY INTO
MEDICAL COLLEGE

Western women's struggle to make inroads into the medical profession had yielded its first and most spectacular success in the United States with the establishment of the Female Medical College of Pennsylvania in 1850. The world's very first college to train women physicians predictably faced considerable hostility from medical men who refused to teach the new students or admit them to the clinic of the local hospitals. Undeterred, the College's first woman dean, Dr Ann Preston, also one of its first graduates, established the adjacent Woman's Hospital of Pennsylvania in 1861. By 1867 the College, located at North College Avenue and Twenty-first Street, was renamed the Woman's Medical College of Pennsylvania (henceforth WMCP), and was already internationally renowned.[1]

WMCP's fame had already reached Anandibai in India to make it her first preference even before arriving in the United States. But her eagerness for the best opportunities was matched by the efforts of competing colleges – the Homeopathic College at New York and the medical college at Boston – to attract the much-publicised 'Hindoo lady'. But it was to Dean Rachel Bodley of WMCP that Mrs Carpenter wrote personally on her ward's behalf on 18 June 1883:

> Dear Madam,
>
> I have in my care Mrs Anandibai Joshee, a Hindoo lady of high caste. She has come to America to study medicine that she might serve her fellow country women in the capacity of surgeon and physician. Hearing from many sources that the Female College of Pennsylvania is the best and most thorough in its main points and believing from some things I have heard and seen in print that steps have already been taken to secure for my ward the advantages of your College, I write to ask you to please inform me what arrangements, if any, have been

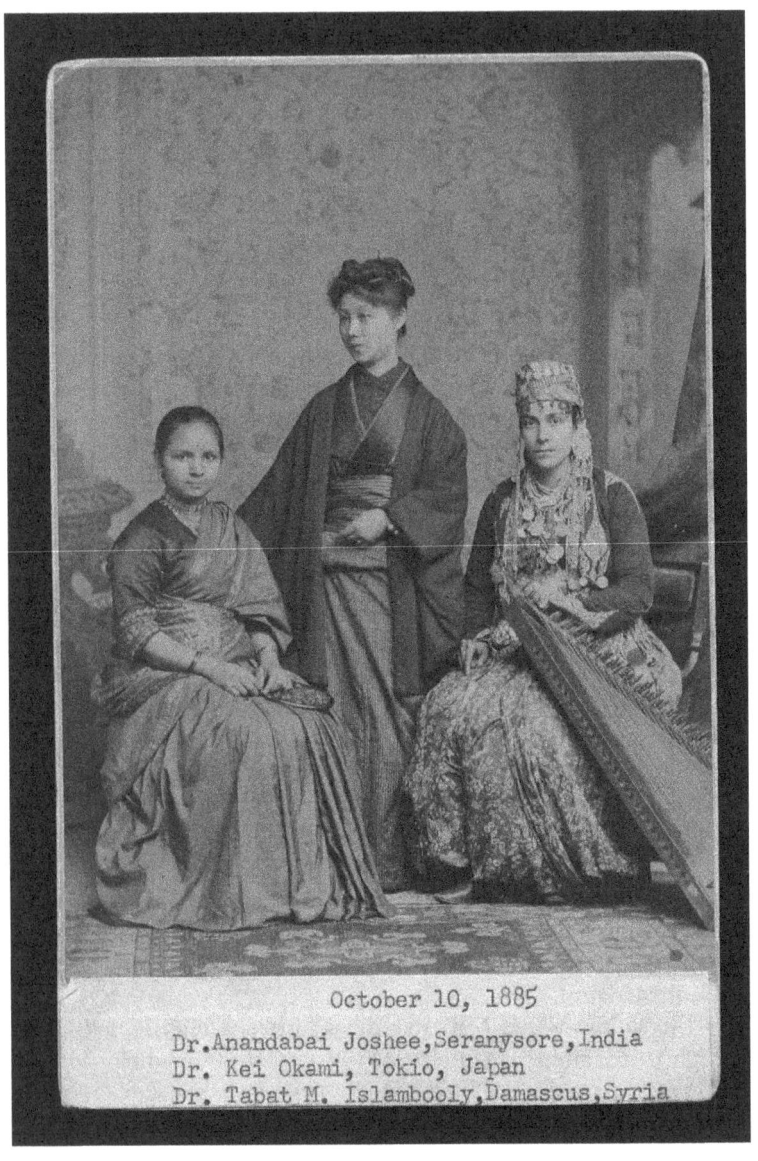

October 10, 1885

Dr.Anandabai Joshee,Seranysore,India
Dr. Kei Okami, Tokio, Japan
Dr. Tabat M. Islambooly,Damascus,Syria

Figure 9.1 Anandibai with a Japanese and a Syrian student of the WMCP

Source: Courtesy of Legacy Center Archives & Special Collections, Drexel University College of Medicine, Philadelphia. http://drexel.edu/LegacyCenter

made. Also if Mrs Joshee would need to attend lectures now, before the close of the term.

If she could begin her studies at home with me and continue them through the summer, taking up as much as you deem necessary for the beginning of a thorough course, without incurring the expense of a trip to Philadelphia before fall, she would prefer to do so. Her means are very limited and the ways to attain the end in view is not yet clear.

We are in correspondence with the Deans of several colleges and shall form plans for Mrs Joshee with care and deliberation. Believing that you or other eminent Philadelphians had already taken an interest in her before her arrival, I feel willing and glad to respect that interest by asking your advice at the outset and what preparations if any have been made for her and what her advantages will be in going to Philadelphia rather than New York.

It would suit our convenience better to have her in the latter city, but we have her best good at heart, and seek only that. Please find enclosed a letter and circular from your friend and mine, Mrs Marlag, MD

A reply at your convenience would greatly oblige.

Yours most respectfully
(Mrs) Theodocia Carpenter[2]

The enclosed letter from Dr Marlag added a personal appeal on behalf of Anandibai, who 'looks very intelligent':

I am doing all in my power to prevent her going to N.Y. to study although some keep holding out such tempting ideas – I beg her to be rather than appear to be a true, earnest, well-educated, intelligent physician and surgeon; and the future of the women of her country depends upon her course here now in the next five years. . . . I feel there is such a grand field for useful work from your college in her country and which a number of your graduates have already toiled in that you will be personally interested in this lady.

Dr Marlag, like Mrs Thoburn in Calcutta, was jealously guarding the College's national and international leadership role in competition with other nearby medical colleges, which also tried to attract Anandibai, especially the Homeopathic College in New York which was about to offer Anandibai a scholarship.[3]

Dean Rachel Bodley (1831–1888) was amenable to these requests. She had been elected to the Chair of Chemistry and Toxicology at the WMCP in 1865 and was the first woman professor of chemistry in the United States on record. In 1874 she was elected dean. A popular teacher able to establish rapport with her students (as evidenced by the affectionate letters of Drs Thoburn and Marlag), she was a single woman who looked after her old mother. She was also known for her 'spirit of hospitality', with which she welcomed into her home 'strangers of many nations'.[4] Dr Bodley was quick to pursue the matter and wrote officially the following morning (19 June 1883) to Mr Alfred Jones, Secretary of the College's Executive Committee, enclosing the letters of Dr Thoburn and Dr Marlag, as well as the article by Mrs Gracey:[5]

Dear Sir,
This morning's mail brings me the first definite intelligence I have rec'd concerning the arrival of Mrs Joshee (the Hindoo lady) in this country.

A half-dozen reporters of the city press representing as many city papers have been calling upon me and writing to me in regard to her, during the last month, so remarkable do they regard her coming to be. . . .

You will observe that Mrs Joshee is a Hindoo, a member of the Brahmo Samaj, the new Hindoo sect. she brings therefore no testimonial (such as our printed rules require) from any missionary society.

Would it be possible for your Committee to perform the graceful act of awarding her a scholarship? This would at once distance all other competing institutions and make her sojourn with us certain. Her talents and learning undoubtedly qualify her for the scholarship.

So much interest is felt in her, through the paragraphs of the reporters that doubtless interest for her medical education can be raised. But if the College in this dignified manner can welcome and provide for the Hindoo – she will not need to become the beneficiary of the public. From what Mrs Carpenter says, I suppose 'half fees' would not be sufficient for her need.

Respectfully,
Rachel Bodley

Dr Bodley's favourable letter indirectly accentuated the Hindoo woman's educational handicap: It appears that Christian women had the advantage of accessing Western educational institutions through the mandatory missionary testimonials. But the disadvantaged Anandibai was fortunate enough in having influential friends and in having generated enough public interest. She added her own partly emotional appeal (on 28 June) while supplying further information and inquiring about possible funding from Mr Alfred Jones, obviously not having yet heard in this regard:

Dear Sir,

I beg to ask, if upon any terms *pecuniarily* consistent with my means, I may be allowed to enter the Woman's Medical College of [Pennsylvania] for a thorough course of study. I have with me seventy dollars and my husband expects to send me twenty dollars per month less the cost of sending.

I was eighteen years of age last month.

I have been once through English Grammar, have studied thorough Arithmetic in my own language and as far as Division in English. . . . I have read the histories of England, Rome, Greece and India.

I have learnt to read and speak in seven [Indian] languages. . . .

Though I may not meet in all points the requirement for entering College, I trust that as my case is exceptional and peculiar, your people will be merciful and obliging. My health is good and this with that determination which has brought me to your country against the combined opposition of friends and caste ought to go a long way towards helping me carry out the purpose for which I came, i.e. to render to my poor suffering countrywomen the true medical aid they so sadly stand in need of and which they would rather die for than accept at the hands of a male physician. The voice of humanity is with me and I must not fail. My soul is moved to help the many who cannot help themselves and I feel sure that God Who has me in His care will influence the many that can and should share in this good work, to lend me such aid and assistance as I may need. I ask nothing for myself individually, but all that is necessary to fit me for my work I humbly crave at the door of your College, or any other that shall give me admittance.

For the kind encouragement already received and the hope held out I feelingly subscribe myself,

Yours gratefully
Anandibai Joshee

The appeal, made on ideological grounds and in the name of the needy women of India, could not fail, especially in view of the number of WMCP graduates who had chosen to work in India. In addition to this Indian connection, the College also had a progressive and international image. After all, the second African American woman to receive a medical degree, Rebecca Cole, had graduated from this very College in 1867.[6] Anandibai would be the first Indian woman to enrol there. Her graduating class of 1886 included a British woman from India and a Russian woman among the thirty-three candidates; her juniors included a Japanese woman and a Turkish woman (see Plate 5). The College was prompt in offering all possible help.

*

Part of the summer, however passed in indecision. Probably at the end of August, Anandibai wrote to Gopalrao:

> No decision has been made so far as to where I am to stay, but it leans heavily in favour of Philadelphia. The Superintendent [Dean] of the College, Miss Bodley, and the Secretary, Mr Jones, are both very kind, and insist that I should be with them. They have made excellent arrangements for everything. A couple of rooms have been obtained for me in a house opposite the College in a good neighbourhood, so that I should not have any problem in the winter when the snow would make it difficult for an inexperienced person to walk. There are also rooms on the fourth floor of the College building itself, but no other students are staying there, so it would be lonely and depressing for me. The above arrangement has been made to avoid that, says the Dean. My three-year course is to cost 600 dollars [about Rs 1,800]. In my application I stated the true facts. The scholarship I am offered is meant for those between the ages of twenty and thirty. But I have completed only eighteen. Even so, I have been awarded the scholarship. Isn't it surprising? I did not reduce my age or increase it. I wrote only the truth. Be that as it may. At the New York College, the Dean and Secretary will award me a freeship and make other arrangements as above. Also, the Dean of the Boston College has invited me with a similar offer. Let's see what happens. The Boston College is quite new. [The] New York College is about 20–22 years old, and the 34-year old Philadelphia College is the oldest and the most reputed. It is well-known for its courses, and surgery is also taught there.

Aunt thinks I should stay with her, but she will do whatever is best for me. So let's see how things turn out. Everything is expensive here. Webster's Dictionary costs 25 rupees! But a gentleman has lent me his own copy; it is the current edition and a very good one. I have 60 dollars with me.[7]

The decision was finally made in favour of WMCP, and the two women paid a visit to Dean Bodley, which remained imprinted in the latter's memory:

[I]n September, 1883, there came to my door a little lady in a blue cotton saree, accompanied by her faithful friend, Mrs B.F. Carpenter . . ., and since that hour, when, speechless for very wonder, I bestowed a kiss of welcome upon the stranger's cheek in lieu of words, I have loved the women of India.[8]

On 10 September, Anandibai informed Gopalrao about her choice of Philadelphia. She was to leave on 27 September, accompanied by Mrs Carpenter.[9]

*

Anandibai's next letter to Gopalrao was sent from Philadelphia on 2 October and reassured him as to her welcome at the College:

Your letter of 13th August arrived last night. I was very happy. I arrived here on the 28*th* with Aunt. We went straight to Dean Bodley's house and both of us stayed there for two days. On the second day the Dean gave me a reception in the evening. It was attended by over five hundred men and women. I was standing between the Dean and Aunt [to receive the guests]. The people here are very nice. I wore the red *pitambar* for the reception.[10]

The reception, an elaborate affair held on 30 September, was reported in the local press, from which it was reproduced by both the *Mahratta* (18 November 1883) and the *Theosophist* (December 1883, Supplement, pp. 39–40):

ANANDA BAI'S RECEPTION
    Greeting to the Brahmin Lady who will become a Philadelphia student
    (Philadelphia Press)

The parlors of Dr Rachel L. Bodley, Dean of the Woman's Medical College, . . . were crowded yesterday afternoon with ladies and gentlemen assembled to meet Mrs Ananda Bye Joshi [sic], a Brahmin lady of Serampore who has come to this country to study medicine . . .

Mrs Joshi, a plump little woman, but eighteen years of age, and of a decidedly brown complexion, stood in the center of the drawing-room, and shook hands with the guests as they were presented. She was dressed in full Native costume for a lady, with the characteristic sari, or silk scarf of Pompeian red, bordered with gold thread, forming the overdress, covering the shoulders and breast, and if necessary, the head. The garment is about ten yards long, and has no fastening . . . underneath the sari, and visible on the left shoulder, was a black silk vest with a V-shaped corsage. The sari was fastened at the breast by a beautiful brooch set with large pearls. In her ears were ornaments of gold filigree, set with pearls, and at her throat were necklaces of gold filigree and pearls. Her bracelets were of jade, a sacred green stone carved into rings.[11] A wreath of jessamine was woven in with her hair, which was jet black, and parted a little on one side. Her hands were encased in kid gloves, so that she could touch the hands of strangers without being contaminated. Between her eyes was a peculiar mark of purple and red paint which denoted the caste of the lady to be a Brahmin.[12]

Mrs Joshi's husband is a prominent member of the Brahmo Samaj, a Progressive Hindu Society of which Ram Mohun Roy was the founder, and Keshub Chunder Sen is the present leader. . . .

Among those present were . . . and many graduates and instructors in the Woman's Medical College.

The report, focusing on details of dress, was obviously authored by a woman, possibly by Mrs Dall, who had spent a few years in Bengal with her missionary husband and who was present on the occasion. Despite its tendency to stress the exotic and its several inaccuracies (all Indian women covering their heads, bangles of the 'sacred jade', and the *kunku* as a caste mark), it succeeded in foregrounding both Anandibai's achievement and the College's cosmopolitan record.

In all probability, Anandibai sent a clipping of the report to Gopalrao who, with his usual alacrity, sent it to the newspapers he was closely acquainted with. The *Theosophist* was predictably incensed at the reference to Gopalrao's membership of the Brahmo Samaj and added an editor's note contesting it.

The local Philadelphia newspapers continued to report on Anandibai's presence as a novelty. The *Philadelphia Inquirer* (5 October 1883) noted with approval that 'the Hindoo woman . . . proposes to take a four years' course' at the WMCP. Other papers, like the *Philadelphia Evening Bulletin* (1 October 1883), found all this publicity unwarranted: '[F]or the life of us we cannot see why a Hindoo doctress should be any more of a lioness than a respectable American woman student'.

*

After the formal reception, Mrs Dall met Anandibai informally as well, and her immediate reaction to Anandibai was couched in clearly racial terms:

> She looks like a stout, dumpy mulatto girl not especially interesting until her yellow face lights up, and light up it did as she gathered from a helping word of mine, that I was familiar with the customs of her people. . . . Her English is exquisite. There is hardly a flaw in pronunciation or construction. If I had not known, I should have thought her born in this country. . . .
>
> Her feeling of caste is still uppermost. She receives her guests with impassive dignity like a true Oriental, and was one of only two or three in her class who chose to stay and see a painful operation for necrosis performed on a young child this week. It was not from indifference, for she spoke of it with painful emotion. She has shown curiosity but once [on meeting a mulatto girl], however much she may have felt it. . . .
>
> When we parted, she put out her hand. 'I feel as if I had found a friend', she said. 'It is the first time anybody has known about me', and then I saw the beauty in the lambent eyes.[13]

*

A whirlwind of activity and excitement carried Anandibai into the Dean's reception, a climactic entry into academic life in Philadelphia; and on 3 October she passed the Matriculation, or entrance, examination to the College and officially embarked on her medical studies.[14] But the aftermath left her acutely homesick and depressed, as the full enormousness of the task confronted her. In her letter of 2 October to

Gopalrao, she concluded her description of the Dean's reception with a personal touch:

> The next morning I completed my toilette, took my leave of the Dean, came to my own house and arranged everything. Aunt helped me to settle in and stayed the night too. In the morning we got up rather early, breakfasted, did some shopping (that is to say, bought some pots and pans) and went straight to the station, reaching just as the train was leaving. As Aunt already had a ticket, she boarded the moving train. Three passengers gave her a hand and lifted her up; by God's grace she boarded safely.
>
> After that I returned home to find total emptiness around me. The thought that nobody dear to me was close by made me burst into tears. I am unable to think. I don't feel like eating or drinking, reading or writing, or even living. In the midst of this your letter arrived, asking me why I cannot rid myself of sloth. It is indeed true that I am lazy, but it is also true that there is a lot of work. The day after tomorrow, College will start, and life will then turn hectic. The college courses appear to be extremely difficult. The current state of my mind cannot be gauged by any but the Almighty God. At Aunt's house I felt completely at home; now I feel as if I am abandoned in a forest. It is true that people here are kind, but I am alone and lost, and find nothing to be agreeable. If I eat anything, it tastes like poison; if I sleep, the bed pricks me like thorns. Yesterday I felt listless and paid a short visit to the Dean. She insisted on my staying the night, but I came home.[15]

Having set up household for herself with great enthusiasm, Anandibai seems to have spent less than a month there. The dual burden of studies and household chores proved impossible to cope with, loneliness became an unwelcome but constant companion, and the smoky coal stove in her room proved to be a great nuisance and a health hazard.[16] By the end of October she moved into Dean Bodley's house, which was to become her home for the rest of her stay in Philadelphia. Later, Dr Bodley herself recalled her dilemma:

> She tried faithfully, this little woman of eighteen, to prosecute her studies, and the same time to keep caste rules and cook her own food; but the anthracite coal stove in her room was a constant vexation, and likewise a source of danger; and the solitude of the individual house-keeping was overwhelming. . . . After a trial of two weeks, her health declined to such an alarming

extent that I invited her to pay a short visit in my home, and she never left it again to dwell elsewhere in Philadelphia during her student residence. In the performance of college duties, going in and out, and up and down, always in her measured, quiet, dignified, patient way, she has filled every room, as well as the stairways and halls, with memories which now hallow the home.[17]

Interestingly, this cross-religious friendship was as problematic for the Christian as it was for the orthodox Hindu, and Bodley's hospitality was not free of anxious moments, as she confided to a colleague who recalled

Mrs Joshee became an inmate of her house . . ., eating and drinking according to the rites of her creed. As an earnest Christian, the Dean debated much with herself as to what her duty was towards Mrs Joshee. But she decided she should have perfect freedom to go where she would and read what she chose, but the Dean once said she felt a terrible responsibility resting on her. Hers was the home the Hindu had chosen and if the observant, shrewd, criticizing nature saw aught of the inconsistency between the precepts of Christ and the practice of his servants living there, it might deter her from accepting Christianity.[18]

Even Bodley's genuine warmth was not entirely untinged by the hope of converting Anandibai to Christianity. In fact, Gopalrao was later to allege that she did indeed try her best to convert Anandibai, though this sounds like his usual exaggerated and wild statements.[19]

*

Concern for his wife propelled Gopalrao to characteristically precipitate action, and once a delay in her letter almost scared him into sending a telegram. As usual, she comforted him with soothing words:

If the pressure of work delays my letters to you, please do not feel anxious. Do not even think of sending a telegram. Rest assured that I am happy wherever I am on the face of this earth. Please do not be careless about your meals. Write and give your news in detail.[20]

These letters exchanged the latest news. In late 1883 she wrote about Pandita Ramabai, who was in England:

A letter has come from Ramabai. Her friend [Anandibai Bhagat who had accompanied her from India] committed suicide.

I feel very sorry for Ramabai. She writes about having lost her hearing due to some illness. The poor woman is beset by calamities. What can she do?[21] I was happy to read the letters in the *Indian Mirror*. I have sent you some newspapers from here. They will arrive duly.[22]

There were also new experiences and discoveries of the American way of life to share:

Aunt's husband has bought me a lovely little clock which is ticking away. It will be very useful for keeping the College timings. It is about five inches tall and three and a half inches broad, and looks compact. The clocks here have an alarm which works like this: on one side of the clock there is a small bowl, the size of a 'ghee' bowl. One sets the alarm for whatever time one wants to wake up, and turns the hand. When the hand reaches that hour, there is a loud ringing sound. I woke up to that sound today. We do not have this facility [in India], and I don't remember having seen it in England.

There is an elevated railroad here, and the underground is planned. In large stores there is a marvellous arrangement for getting from one floor to another. Anybody who wishes to avoid aching feet from climbing up seven flights of stairs can use it. This is how it works: on one side of the store.[23](in the same building) there is an empty space the size of a small room, which is walled in from the first floor to the last. Into this empty space is fitted a small room, held by very strong ropes on all sides, and with some chairs inside. One can go up or down to any floor one wants without even feeling it move. What a wonderful convenience!

As a rare account of the American experience, Anandibai's letters had a definite popular interest which Gopalrao was quick to exploit by getting them newspaper publicity. *Kesari* published some excerpts, prefacing them with a by now predictable comment on the polarity between Anandibai and Pandita Ramabai:

Mrs Anandibai Joshee's character is very different from Pandita Ramabai's. We strongly hope that this humble and well-behaved lady will acquire a good training in medicine as planned, and, without committing any lapse with regard to religion and conduct as the Sanskrita [Ramabai] did, return to this country and work for the welfare of her destitute countrywomen in many ways. Those who have personally seen Mrs Anandibai recount that her temperament is not fickle, obstinate, or arrogant, but very submissive and deferential. Anandibai's letters give ample evidence of her faith in God, fear of sin, and love for her husband, and also contain important suggestions about trade, etc. we have made arrangements to give some news of Anandibai every now and then, as long as she stays in America. In today's issue we present some passages from her letters, which we hope will greatly interest the readers.[24]

The excerpts were followed by a reiteration of good wishes: 'We hope that Anandibai will return safely after completing her studies in four years, and utilises her hard-earned knowledge in the cause of national welfare'.

Thus, Anandibai was installed as the icon of the new Indian womanhood – a 'submissive and deferential' *pativrata* who observed the necessary religious rites and whose movements could be monitored through her letters and who was watched over by the trustworthy Mrs Carpenter. This offered a contrast to Ramabai on all points – Ramabai, who stayed with Christian nuns and whose conversion to Christianity soon created shockwaves.

*

The thought of a long separation was unbearable, and Anandibai continued to miss her husband acutely. Possibly around this time, she wrote

> please try as hard as possible to come here. It is difficult to continue living apart much longer! . . . If you have no money, I will send the few jewels I have; or if you want money, I will sell them here and send you the money. Together they will certainly cover your fare.[25]

Letters from friends and well-wishers also poured in. To one such letter from an eminent Maharashtrian lady friend (possibly Ramabai Ranade), Anandibai replied in Marathi on 2 November 1883:

> My very dear sister . . .
> Your letter filled with good wishes came yesterday. I am unable to describe the joy I felt at the sight of it. I am very grateful to you for taking the trouble to write. I hope that the correspondence will always continue. Despite my desire to write to everybody and give my news, I have to act contrary to my

wishes due to a heavy load of work. For the same reason, I have
not received any news from Panditabai for a month; the fault
is not hers but mine. She and her dear daughter are well. In
her last letter she wrote about the sad demise of her friend. You
must have heard the news too.

Obviously Anandibai had not yet heard about Ramabai's conversion.

I was very much delighted by your interesting account of the
Arya Mahila Samaj. The Samaj was established before I left
India, but I did not know much about it, because I was in
Calcutta. It gives me great pleasure and satisfaction to know
that it is doing well. As it is primarily a women's association,
and also established by a woman, I am very proud of it. Who
would not feel admiration for the burning desire of one's fellow
countrywomen to obtain their rights? I pray to God Almighty
to let it always prosper.

Anandibai then goes on to describe her college life. The WMCP was
the best among the medical colleges in the United States, attended by
women from all over the world. The reception given by the Dean in
her honour was attended by about one hundred people, including the
College faculty and officials, as well as other doctors, so that she felt she
was among friends.

The semester had started in early October, and Anandibai had taken
the six first-year subjects: chemistry, physiology, anatomy, materia med-
ica, surgery, and histology. She took copious notes in class. During the
second year these subjects would be continued and four more added.
Her plan was to complete the college course in three years and spend
the fourth year in a women's hospital. *After four years I intend to return
to my homeland and put my original plan into practice. This is my dream;
it is up to God to fulfil it'.* Towards this end, she studied whenever she
found the time. She rested seven to eight hours, spent two hours on
letter-writing, an hour and a half on meals, half an hour on visits, half
an hour on her toilette, and the rest of the time on lectures and studies.
There were many letters to write: The day before she had received seven
letters!

There was no change in her diet. Her dress, however, had changed:
She wore the sari Gujarati style, so that she could wear warm clothes;
the Maharashtrian style of draping the nine-yard sari exposed the legs
slightly, which was to be avoided, in view of the cold climate. She
always covered her head while outside, and also draped a shawl over

her shoulders. She found this Indian dress to be better than the English dress. None bothered her about her dress, as they had done during her brief sojourn in England and Ireland. In Cork she had been practically mobbed. The Americans were 'very affectionate, kind and friendly'. Anandibai also religiously wore her kunku, bangles, and mangalsutra.

> My obstinacy about retaining my national costume is because I want to be different from others; secondly, it is a symbol of one's motherland; and thirdly, I do not like the English 'dresses'. This does not mean that I am aloof from these people; on the contrary, they want me to dress in this fashion.

Anandibai's experiments with cooking for herself did not last long, in view of her hectic schedule. So, the previous week she had moved to the Dean's house, and her meals consisted of chapatis and lentils.

She mentions the two Maharashtrians she had encountered at Roselle: Guruji and Rajwade, and expressed strong disapproval for the latter's lack of manners, which might prejudice Americans against Indians.

> The American people are very ignorant about India. (This used to hurt me in the beginning.) They even doubt whether our houses have windows! They see no difference between India and Africa! The wisest among them are the missionaries who have returned from India! But even their knowledge is limited. They come back here and frighten everyone with the weapon of 'idolatry'. In addition, they have discovered our two weaknesses: 'child marriage' and 'widow remarriage'. But even so, they hardly understand the real problem. It is to be hoped that this ignorance of theirs will soon disappear; but until such time there is the possibility of their misunderstanding us. Therefore it *behooves* everyone to be careful. I feel proud to mention that the Bengali gentleman Babu Protap Chunder Mazumdar has received much acclaim here.[26]

*

At the end of 1883, Anandibai wrote to G. H. (Bapusaheb) Ketkar, Gopalrao's first wife's brother and the couple's friend:

> The account of [Pandita] Ramabai, if true, is very saddening. She has really brought a stigma to female education, religious faith, Truth, etc. It is difficult to assess the extent to which it will obstruct female education; but it will certainly not leave

the numerous efforts in that direction unaffected. Last week a newspaper here published the news that Ramabai was the guest of Max Mueller. This suggests that the rumour of conversion is not true. Scholars do not pay much attention to religious matters, and that news is fresh. . . .

These days I am with the Dean of the College, and think that I will stay on here. This lady is aged and very industrious. She loves me dearly. Bapusaheb, I am neither alone, nor in a strange country. All people love me dearly. I do not at all feel that I am in a foreign country. All people are ever ready to help me. Even the laundress charges me less, and not more. (I mention this as an example.) I have a home wherever I go. People do not make fun of me. Even small children are polite. I am under such an obligation to the American people, that I have no hope of ever repaying them. The reason why they do so much is not that I am good, but that they are good. They are generous and good-hearted, and act accordingly. Please do not worry about me at all. You have done a great deal for me. May this kindness always continue.

Anandibai then describes the large residential college for destitute boys built by Girard, adjacent to the WMCP. The good upbringing, education, and vocational skills provided there had reclaimed many boys from a life of poverty, sloth, and crime. Anandibai rues the fact that no such institution existed in India.[27]

One of Anandibai's last letters of the year (6 December) was addressed to Gopalrao:

Tomorrow it will be exactly eight months since we parted. My mind has been so involved in studies that I feel as if I have just arrived. Time will continue to pass equally fast, and we will soon meet again.

In your last letter you wielded your pen sharply against your female cook, as common people often do. You have also mentioned briefly how you rebuke her. I already know that women from Kashi [Banaras] are immoral. And truly it is a shameful thing. But this is not creditable behavior. . . . talking about xxx you have said that, 'women are all alike!' Perhaps you did not realise what you said, but it certainly broke my heart. Is there no difference? After all, Sita and Chandrasena were contemporaries. Poor and helpless indeed are women – they fall prey to temptation and are despised. Their condition is so vile as to arouse pity, but nobody pays any heed to them. When they become destitute and diseased, people do not allow them to approach them, and do not even cast a covetous glance at them! When they are doing well, people praise their beauty, and that is what causes their downfall later. Then they acquire evil habits and are immediately reduced to starvation and begging at the doors of the same evil, licentious people who originally led them down the immoral path! Instead of rescuing these women from that state, they abuse them and drive them away. May God have mercy on them! Even the thought of their destitution makes my heart tremble, and I begin to wonder why I was ever born if I am so powerless to rescue them! O you unfortunate creatures, this world will not liberate you, but on the contrary, revile you. Death alone will emancipate you. . . .

. . . A man may marry one woman, bind another with promises, bring a third to live with him, and, after all this, plan to betroth a fourth. And, without having any greater rights than his wife, mother or sister, he may say that he has leave to do what he will! What a tragic state of affairs! The more I think about it, the more it pains me. Truly, this thought has penetrated my heart deeply. You yourself may ask how many families he [someone mentioned earlier] has ruined for the satisfaction for his immoral amorous designs. You will find any number of such men! They are strongly swayed by this immoral desire and are powerless to conquer it. In fact, real bravery and glory lie in subjugating it rather than in submitting to it. It is a far easier matter to conquer an enemy than to conquer immoral desire. I feel great pity for the poor people who are controlled by such desire because they are very ignorant and foolish. And the women are not usually the guilty ones, only entrapped. . . .

. . . I make you one request, that you should take pity on your cook. She is good, and you say that she keeps the house in better order than I do. She also has feelings of pleasure and pain, as you do. So please retain her for my sake, and try to reform her. I have already told you how this can be done. . . .

In one matter I need a little help from you, which you will surely give. During the next summer vacation, I want to give a talk. What topic should I select? I think, 'Indian women' is a good subject. There must have appeared a lot of articles in newspapers; please send them and other information also.

Your letter has just arrived – don't make me suffer like this. Remember clearly that God is concerned about us. Ramabai is not Anandibai, and Anandibai is not Ramabai! The two are different individuals, created for different work. Even if I die, I will not act contrary to my beliefs. Ramabai is twenty times more learned than I. (There is no similarity at all between us.) just as the marsh grass bends but does not break, I have made a resolve in this regard. . . . why do people suspect me? I don't understand how I have erred. I am not at all affected by people's anger, hatred, or vileness. It stays in my mind just as long as a drop of water remains on a lotus leaf.

Regarding his plans to go to America and the possibility of a business venture, Gopalrao had consulted some eminent but unenthusiastic people about whom Anandibai waxes sarcastic:

Rao Bahadur xxx's letter is too full of advice. . . . these people are just too intelligent for poor hapless India. There is no hope that India can escape from them. They are submerged in hollow pride. I feel bad that you consulted them about such a matter. Be patient. If God has concern for us, He has surely made some arrangement for us. And, after four years, I myself will make some arrangement for you, I think. Don't show my letters to any such person. . . . keep [them] with yourself. Or else, burn them as soon as you have done with them. You are too altruistic for this world, and would get no reward for it except abuse and disrespect! Until I get through my studies (or my studies get through me), I am unable to finalise anything. . . . The day should have been longer than it is, to provide more time. . . . And if I start spending my time in this manner, how will I retain my first rank in the class?

This is the only indication of the important fact of Anandibai's academic success.

I have not written to the Rani of Baroda as advised by that gentleman. . . . It is better to wait until [the proper time]. . . .
This letter has been written partly in an easy chair and partly in bed, because I am a little unwell. There is no cause for anxiety. I am near a doctor, but am not taking any medicine. I think this due to a change of weather and will be cured without medicine. . . . It could also be the result of physical or mental stress. . . . Our ancient Hindu medical science recommends

that no medicine should be taken for the first three days. This will show you how wise and perfect our science is.

P.S. I am sending a photograph of myself taken by Prof. Bodley. Everybody sends namaskar (salaams) to you.[28]

Notes

1 In 1970 the WMCP became the coeducational Medical College of Pennsylvania (MCP); *Guide to Collections* in the Archives and Special Collections on Women in Medicine; MCP Archives.

2 Copies from the original letter in the Archives of the Woman's Medical College, available in the Bombay University Library.

3 Dall, p. 101.

4 Croasdale 1888.

5 From the MCP Archives, available in Bombay University Library.

6 The Guide to Collections, p. 9.

7 *Kesari*, 6 November 1884.

8 Bodley, p. i.

9 *Kesari*, 6 November 1883.

10 Kanitkar, p. 172, my translation.

11 The jade bangles cannot be explained.

12 The 'kunku' has often been construed as a caste mark in the West.

13 Dall, p. 116.

14 Ibid, p. 101.

15 Kanitkar, p. 172.

16 In the popular Maharashtrian mind, this coal stove was the only reason for her final illness.

17 Bodley, p. ii.

18 Croasdale 1888.

19 Kanitkar, p. 270.

20 Ibid, p. 174, my translation; date of letter not known.

21 Pandita Ramabai had left for England also in April 1883, along with her little daughter and Anandibai Bhagat, to study medicine. But the discovery of her incurably defective hearing ruled this out. During this difficult time, Anandibai Bhagat committed suicide for fear of being converted to Christianity by force. For details, see Meera Kosambi, 'Introduction,' in *Pandita Ramabai in Her Own Words*, Delhi: Oxford University Press, 2000.

22 *Kesari*, 6 November 1883, my translation.

23 Ibid.

24 Ibid.

25 Kanitkar, p. 212, my translation.

26 Ibid, pp. 182–83, my translation.

27 Ibid, p. 192, my translation.

28 Ibid, p. 229, my translation.

10

LIFE IN PHILADELPHIA, EARLY 1884

The year 1884 dawned even as Anandibai was struggling to balance her new life with her old.[1] The heavy college schedule occasionally became even more difficult because of a personal loss. The sudden death of a woman doctor who had been kind to her led her to philosophise on the human condition:

> Is she taken from those who love her dearly and need her so badly? What a mystery this world is! Happy today, miserable tomorrow! How true that our deepest sorrows flow from our deepest affections. What an instrument of torture one's own heart is!

The news from India was not always pleasant. An inimical letter she received on 4 January distressed her so deeply that her 'face was clouded by indignation' and her friends thought she was sick, when she received another of her occult visions:

> All at once a beautiful young lady with a sweet voice came and sat down by me, and pressing my hand with her own, said: 'Dear child, do not [be despondent]. Providence is just and merciful, and means you no harm. Have courage to endure many more such things. Do you not remember how I was persecuted in the presence of my husband, the king? Be true and faithful'. Then she seemed to disappear. I felt her presence though I could no longer see her, and was comforted.[2]

*

Anandibai's regular and copious correspondence with Gopalrao reflected the ups and downs of what had obviously been a stormy marriage. On 9 January she wrote probably her first letter of the year to him:

Your fourth letter came today. I had a slight fever yesterday and feel weak. Doctor [Bodley?] told me not to go out. I am not too ill, so please do not worry. I am a little exhausted because of the rain, snow, cold, studies, and such other things. Everything is covered by snow today. In some places, there is 30 inches of snow and the temperature has dropped below zero. I have not suffered much from the snow yet; I take great precautions. I have no problems about food at all. There will be no change in my condition, no matter where I am on the face of this earth. These days I am with the Dean. I had already informed you of this.

Gopalrao had taken instant exception to Anandibai's change of dress, which he discovered from her photos. She reasoned patiently with him, as usual:

I will be satisfied only with an Indian costume. All the women look at my dress and say, 'It will be so delightful if the Indian dress comes into fashion next'. The Maharashtrian dress will be comfortable only in the summer and I feel it would be improper to change my costume [according to season], besides looking like a performer in different guises. I have resolved to keep the same manner of dress all the time. As soon as I leave this country, I will dress in the Maharashtrian style; that is my firm decision. I did not wear the nose ring every day even in India, then why is it surprising if I do not do so now? Is this to be taken to mean that I have given up wearing it forever? Oh, that is grand indeed! . . .

. . . Prin. xxx's letter is very insipid. And that is not to be wondered at. When you write to him, please thank him and inform him that my plan is unchanged. One must expect people to have doubts about me because of Ramabai.

The houses here have rooms much smaller than ours. There is nothing remarkable about them. The floors are covered with beautiful grass mats in the summer and carpets in the winter. The bedsteads are nothing special. Some houses have stoves in the basement, so that the whole house is nicely warmed. In others there are fireplaces in the walls. From inside the house, the rain and snow present a strange scene. The snow does not make a sound like the rain, it falls lightly and gently like a feather. It is white like powdered sugar. But when the rain falls on the snow, it becomes ice which looks exactly like glass. If it remains in the streets by mistake, people fall heavily and hurt themselves badly. The Government rule is that every house owner must clear the portion in front of his gate. So, one has to go outside the city to see the real beauty of Nature. But in order to see human scorn for it, one must visit a city like New York. When I visited Aunt during the vacation, I really enjoyed the grandeur of Nature. One day we all played with snowballs, and I went with Aunt for a ride in the wheel-less carriage called the 'sleigh'. I hope you will not envy me for all this!

There is a lot written about me in the newspapers here. But how can I manage to see it all? In the letter which came last week, you have written about your intention of publishing in book form a collection of all my letters and all the newspaper accounts about me. I know that your motives are pure, but I do not think it would be proper. It will look quite ridiculous. There are those who speak well of me, but there are just as many, or more, who speak ill of me. Moreover, whatever we do is not for show. Nobody would stop us from showing off, but what purpose would it serve? Those who think it right may certainly do so; but not we. We have not made ourselves ridiculous so far. I pray to God that this continues to be so. What is the use of spending one's time and energy on something so meaningless? Please forgive me for writing this. If you find my letters difficult to read, I have no objection to your copying them in a notebook. But I request you not to publish them.

One does not know whether Anandibai was aware of the several long extracts Gopalrao had already had published in newspapers.

There is absolutely no consistency in your letters. Once you wrote that I need not write a long letter but send at least a postcard every week. Another time you wrote that frequent letters are not necessary, but one long letter should be written every month. New instructions all the time! . . . [I]n today's letter you have said: 'If one travels anywhere, one feels the desire to communicate the novelty to those close to one. But for you it makes no difference whether you are in America or even beyond. The people who come here from those parts write large volumes, then why are our people [you] like this? You too must have realised this difference'. Like other people, I too am strongly impressed by the variety of Nature. But there are other subjects which attract me even more strongly like a magnet, day and night. Being inherently phlegmatic, I am not easily swayed. Because of just this one gift, I never lose my independence. After every other step and every other word, I have the refrain, 'What is my duty?'; and my conduct is governed by the decisions I make myself. The fact that I do not describe the things in this country cannot be attributed to my indifference to the beauty of Nature.

. . . I feel that I have undertaken a very hazardous enterprise and bear a great responsibility. I must think far ahead before taking every single step. It is not that someone has thrust this responsibility on me, but I have accepted it willingly. All my happiness is concentrated in it.

Please don't send me anything from there, not even shoes. Send only books if I ask for them. I already have saris. Aunt has given strict instructions that nothing should be sent for the girls. Whatever you send for my expenses should be sent in Aunt's name. If you feel compelled to send me something, then send me a pin which I need for the loose [necks of] blouses I wear these days, as you will see from the photograph I have sent. In England Mrs Johnson bought me one. (I did not ask for it.) I used to wear it all the time, but its three sharp corners used to hurt and scratch me. Now that I will be dissecting, it will not do to have scratches; therefore Aunt has taken it away and said she would never return it. She intends to send it to you to be given away. What concern! Now I have no pin and would not like to wear one made here. I have written this at Aunt's insistence. The pin is worn not as an ornament, but to make the blouse fit snugly around the throat. . . . If it has a space (at the back) for a photograph, insert your photograph there. If it has a locket, I will keep a lock of Aunt's hair in it.

I think Bapusaheb [Ketkars'] advice should be followed. Aunt's thinking and my own is that your departure should be postponed. After I pass my [final] examination, I will join a hospital; you should come during that year so that we can both see this country and return together. This arrangement will be very convenient. I think that Aunt will also write to you. . . . Be patient, it is no use getting restless. One should not do anything impulsively. Please do not resign; do not leave your job.

In the winter, the gardens have no trees with any leaves on them (except a species called Evergreen). Wherever you look, you see only bare branches. A creeper covered by snow, if drenched by the rain, looks just like a glass creeper. It looks as if the central stalk is coated with an overlay of ice, or the creeper is placed inside a glass tube.[3]

The next letter to Gopalrao was a lengthy one, started at the end of January and completed over a week.

Monday [28 January 1884]: Today appears to be a lovely day. For the last several days the weather had turned bad and the streets were slippery. But today everything looks bright and clean. Fresh sparkling snow has started to fall. Fortunately it is thick enough to cover the dirty sidewalks. . . . [T]he sun has taken it upon itself to gladden everyone with its brilliant rays. Even more importantly, I have received a letter from a person whom I love dearly. As I was happily walking to College through the snow, I felt keenly that you should have been here to share this experience. And just as I started to wonder why you were not here, I remembered that it was not in your hands! My eyes were dazzled by the bright sunlight on the snow, and I felt like bottling the snow and sending it immediately for you to see! I think it would be wonderful to have snow on the 4*th* of July in this country, and on hot days at Bombay, Calcutta and other places in India, which seem unending. You will laugh at my writing this. But I cannot bear that intense heat and feel as if I am dying! Now it is almost time to go to College, so I cannot write much more. Until my examination is over, I will not be able to write to you so frequently, because it will disturb my studies. Still, my mind is always filled with thoughts of you.

Thursday, 31*st* [January]: The weather has turned bad again. Leaving the house is out of the question. There is so much fog, rain, dampness, cold, etc. Rain has dirtied the clean snow and made all the streets so slippery that walking has become a calamity! One of my friends at School slipped on the ice and hurt herself so badly; it has become a daily occurrence. Sometimes the girls have themselves to blame, because being either foolish or careless, they don't wear rubber boots which make their legs look fat. Not that the ones who wear boots don't fall, but the chances are fewer. During the whole week, Thursday is the most difficult for us. Not a minute is free during the twelve hours (from 9 a.m. to 9 p.m.)! We are constantly busy, almost like honeybees. . . . A group of college girls can be seen hurrying towards the porch at about 8:30 in the morning, and hastening homewards in the evening. This is our college routine.

It cannot be called happy! Yesterday I wanted you to be with me to walk together happily through the snow, but not today. I want you to share only my happiness, not my unhappiness. I know that you are in a good climate. I want you to have nothing but good things, excellent climate, congenial company. I am prepared to endure all my sufferings alone, as long as I have my happiness only when I am with you. I prefer to suffer unhappiness myself rather than to see others suffer.

Snow teaches us such an excellent lesson; it falls so lightly, without thunder or lightning. Besides it makes all the surroundings as clean and lovely as itself. It treats everybody equally. Is this not a lesson in itself? . . . In fact, it is a model for all to follow. . . .

Saturday [2 February]: Many people feel comfortable in warm weather, and so do you, I think.

Your letter tells me that your quarrel with 'J' [Mr James] continues as before. You know well that I despise impatience, and so I always feel anxious about you because of your usual impulsiveness. If I were in your place, I would conduct myself with greater patience. When you are calm, you are extremely calm. But once your mood changes, it is impervious even to the weight of considered opinion! . . . One should follow the truth and not allow anything in the world to obstruct it. There is nothing more valuable than the truth. Even God likes Truth and its followers. . . . Surely you remember the beautiful maxim, 'Truth alone shall triumph'. . . .

Sunday [3 February]: What a charming view of the sunset sky is visible from the window!! The bright golden sun rays look so lovely against the completely clear sky! Truly this day seems delightful! How happy I feel because I am here! As you cannot come here, I include a brief mention of it in this letter which will leave by tomorrow's mail.

On the 7th of December, I had a dream which I will tell you. . . . I don't understand its significance. I have interpreted it to mean that people will continue to harbour suspicion and prejudice about me until 7th June, but not after that date. Or that I will die on that day. Let us wait and see what happens. But please keep this confidential, won't you?

Please send information about contracting small pox and not about inoculation against it. . . . The best way is to write to the Public Medical Reporter of the Medical General. Please send whatever old and new reports are available there. . . .

One of my friends has asked you to send some books for her and promised to pay me the price here. This anonymous friend is none other than Prof. Bodley herself. The books wanted are the following:

The First Sanskrit Book – one copy
The Second Sanskrit Book – one copy
Sanskrit Dictionary – two copies.

I have not re-read this letter for lack of time. I have written whatever came to my mind. Forgive me if you do not like it, and remember that while I was writing I meant well. . . . I have written to Mr J [James].

Anandibai mentioned being unwell while concluding the letter; this was to flare into a major illness, and her next letter to Gopalrao (dated 19 to 21 February) was written while she was convalescing:

I feel grateful that I am well enough to write to you today. For the first time in two weeks I am holding a pen in my trembling hand. Since my last letter, I was on furlough. Aunt told me she had already informed you that I have been ill. There was no cause for anxiety, but Prof. Bodley admitted that she was really afraid at the time. I felt no fear and she showed none. The slightest sore throat can lead to a real illness in this country, which is why my good friend was so anxious. I am really grateful for her unselfish friendship and the care she bestowed on me. I am unable to describe it. It was to you that my last letter was written and I remember ending it with the words, 'I do not feel well today'. As soon as I completed it, I developed a severe headache. But I thought it was due to over-exertion that morning. A couple of minutes later, when I sat down to eat, I sensed that my throat was hurting and my feet were cold. I was sitting near the stove thinking about this, when Prof. Bodley told me to go and lie down. I went and had a short nap. But on waking up I had such a painful throat that I was unable to eat or drink. It was inflamed, and so I had fever and headache. For eight days I subsisted only on milk. You must have realised the nature of this illness. It is called 'Diphtheria'. My college friends sent me fruit, flowers, letters and ornamental plants every day. There was an experienced woman to nurse me through this illness. The Doctor also visited a few times a day – she is a professor in our College and is very nice. Her name is Dr Brumall. I am surprised that I recovered so quickly. I think the real medicines were my friends' concern, your sweet letter last week, and the daily mail from Roselle. Although my body was aching (even now I am weak) my mind was quite at ease, because I had full faith in God and was certain that He had me under His care. He is my Father, my Mother, my Guide, also my Comforter and my Saviour. This feeling gave me such comfort and joy as I have never before felt during an illness. I will always pray to Him and express my gratitude for this. There are some things I want to tell you, but I will not write them here. I will tell you myself, because they are confidential and I want them to remain so. From the 4th to the 15th I was confined to my bed. I could dress myself and occasionally sit in a chair, but the Doctor had advised me against it until my throat was completely healed. On the 16th I just sat in my room. On the 17th I went to the Library as usual. I feel good if I learn something new. Although I have not started attending College, I will start reading at home after I finish this letter and write one to Aunt. I am feeling refreshed today although I have not yet recovered my strength.[4]

The attack of diphtheria had left Anandibai quite weak, though she tried to resume her daily routine as soon as possible. On 26 February she wrote to Gopalrao:

Two of your letters have arrived. I have decided to answer both. . . . I am going to discuss separately each one of the points in your letter.

First, I beg you not to pay any attention at all to the form of my letters.

Second, you have written that I should forget my intention of returning [to India], and I do not think this is right. It is true that I want for nothing here; the people love me dearly; I have enough for my expenses. (Not just enough, but ample. What you have sent is still intact. After paying directly for the tickets to school, fees, etc., there is a small balance left.) But I cannot complete the task for which I came or discharge my duty by staying here. There is a glut of women doctors here; many think it better not to have them at all, or at least not so many. Men hate them. What is the use of staying in a country where one cannot be so useful? It is not that I was happier in India. Only from you have I received true happiness. You never hurt me with bad language. You ensured my welfare as far as possible.

I was not tormented as other wives were. I used to feel that I was the only happy person in the world. In sum, all my happiness was concentrated in you. It was not my fate to receive happiness from my mother or sisters. Who can help that? If a woman does better than her neighbours, they are bound to be upset. In their view, whoever does better is deceitful. But I am not concerned with such things. I will persevere in doing whatever I have decided to do in spite of all obstacles – this is my firm resolve. To give up now would be undesirable. I was a little sad to hear your decision not to return if you came here. I am indeed very happy here. Do not think that I am in a foreign country. I am in my parental home. No country is foreign to me. All are my brothers and sisters. My only sorrow is your absence. That will vanish if you come, and all will be perfect happiness. But this will be reversed if you do not change your decision, for I shall certainly return. . . . Then what happiness will you enjoy here by yourself? (But how foolish of me to think that your happiness will be affected by my absence.) If your decision is irrevocable, then it would be better if you cancel your trip instead of coming here for four years and staying on. I will somehow manage to pull on for the next four years. I have not lost courage, so don't worry. If you are willing to retract your words and are prepared to come here to see the country and return with me, then please come as soon as you get the opportunity. Your arrival will not disturb my studies. Nothing in the world can distract one from studies, I think.

Third, if you make your home here, what kind of example will you set to the people there [in India]? Will it not be one of selfishness? And that is neither approved nor respected by the virtuous.[5] It is considered to be a vice, which is why you should not be contaminated by it. You should be associated with philanthropy which is counted as a virtue. (Surely you yourself feel this too, but have written otherwise so that I should continue to remain here and be happy – I am convinced of this.) The right place to set a good example is neither America nor any country other than India. Let our people think what they will, I am not concerned. I consider this [plan] to be right, and so do you.

Fourth, I and everybody else are now hopeful of my being able to obtain my MD diploma in three years. God willing, I will then spend one year practising in a women's hospital, and return after completing this four-year training.

Anandibai's next letter to Gopalrao, dated 2 March 1884, was enormously long and traversed a vast terrain:[6]

Your letter of 4*th* January came on time. It was so long and loving that my heart was submerged in happiness. I felt glad to see your determination to endure all calamities and difficulties with courage. Your letter of last week had caused me a great deal of anxiety which was completely erased by this letter. Like a weary traveller in the mid-day heat, I feel refreshed at the sight of the cool shade offered by your letter. The stream in this shade is the contents of your letter, poured straight from your heart, and it alone sustains my life. I feel such an intense desire to meet you, and my mind is so filled with thoughts of you, that I completely lose consciousness of the reality that you are far away beyond the wide ocean. . . .

I feel truly ashamed of my last letter. I now realise that I might have used some very harsh words; but there is no help now. Although they were not used with the intention of hurting you, I fear that they might give you such an impression. I cannot understand how I was able to write them. And, because I cannot write well, it would have been far better had I not written at all. It would be a good thing if, by luck, the letter should be lost. I will never ask your forgiveness for having reminded you of past events. I deserve punishment and am prepared to accept whatever punishment you mete out to me. You know what your wife is like. You know her better than this pen does, and your firm opinion surely tells you what I am like.

There is nothing so humiliating in this world as the realisation of one's wickedness. . . . Do I not know you and your opinion of women? And have I not had personal experience of these? And is it possible to even imagine that I will ever forget them? . . . The other day I happened to attend a gathering here. Some of the women said, 'Anandibai's husband is really much superior to our husbands'. Then another woman said, 'My husband is a businessman. If he even feels that I might learn a profession and be more successful than he, he will never allow me to learn it'. Immediately a third woman said, 'my husband is quite willing, but I myself cannot manage it'. Of course they did not say these things to me, but I overheard them. And indeed I feel proud that I have a husband like yourself. But enough of this mutual admiration. Self-congratulation is sure to put an end to everything else.[7]

Eventually, spousal rivalry was also to sear the Joshees' relationship, but Anandibai had no inkling of it at this time.

A series of sad events were reported in the letter which reached Anandibai in January 1884: the news of Ramabai's conversion, the death of Swami Dayanand Saraswati in October 1883, and the death of the Raja of Kolhapur. Anandibai continues the letter in a philosophical vein:

I felt somewhat relieved at the news of the death of the poor Raja of Kolhapur. In fact this should be considered a happy and not a sad event, because the wretched man has escaped this indescribable suffering and found happiness. When he left this earthly body, his suffering and torment ended. He has gone to a place where there is no distinction of colour, caste, age or profession. Truly it must be a better place than Ahmadnagar or Kolhapur, where the poor man is happy, looked after by kind people who would not subject him to whipping and other torture. He is free from the pain and trouble of this world. Why then should we weep for him? . . .

If Ramabai's religious conversion is motivated by anything other than an error of judgement or a desire for material help, my tongue or pen will never utter a word against her, because I sympathise with those who act upon their conviction and words. That is why I would have been proud of her brave deed and surprised at her courage. But many doubt whether this is indeed the case. . . . Man appears to have three kinds of religious paths which . . . [successively] lead us to increasingly higher states: [Pantheism, Trinitarianism and Monotheism].[8] . . . Love is the bond which holds all people together. This is the secret of all religions, the fraternity of mankind. . . .

You know already that I have made up my mind. All my arguments are finished. . . . Although I do not know what will happen next, I cherish great hope. I will never neglect my duty. If you wish, you can help any country other than India; but I do not understand why one should leave a full plate to go begging elsewhere. Of course I need not tell you that I harbour no prejudice against any country on this earth, but the argument in India's favour is that if God wills me to be useful to my fellow creatures, it is more probable that I should do so in India. I am familiar with our customs and practices; I know our women's way of life better than foreign women do; I also know their religious prohibitions and share the same language. If it is Divine Will to deny Hindu women a medical college, then

I am determined to teach them at least elementary knowledge of health. If need be, I will spare the time for public or private lectures. Let anybody who is bent on harassing me do so. I care for neither praise nor slander. I may feel sorry if my actions are not approved, but I will not abandon my effort. The more I see people's unfavourable side, the more will my determination grow. I draw only encouragement from all quarters. . . .

Bhau [Gopalrao's brother?] agrees with you that he should settle down abroad, and I approve of that. If done wisely, it will undoubtedly be very beneficial. . . . Your words, 'We should introduce reform while remaining Hindu in our customs and practices as we are', are very good and praiseworthy. But please don't say that you despise certain things, because that would not lead to any reform. . . . we ourselves have hated and been hated. This contagious disease has spread widely in India these days. Enough of that hatred now, because it disrupts our future work.

After I entered College, a woman who was an atheist became a theist! Although I do not talk about religion unless compelled to, I thought that this opportunity should not be missed. . . .

There is an Englishwoman in my class who is a close friend of mine. (She calls me sister.) Her history is very sweet. . . . [She has descended from a marriage between a lord attached to the East India Company and an aristocratic Indian woman.] She feels very proud of having at least some connection with Aryans. She started to love me as soon as she saw me. So did I. . . . She proposes to go to India. She is the right person to help me in my work, being highly qualified.

I feel really surprised at the ignorance of these [American] people. They ask such childish and foolish questions regarding child marriage, that it really annoys me. They ask so many things that I have never even heard or seen in my life. Recently we had a visit from a lady doctor who is, or is considered to be, learned and knowledgeable. She was requested by our American Medical Association to draw up a questionnaire on 'Women Doctors for India'. Printed questions have been sent to women doctors in India, and have been given to me also although I am not a doctor. I will answer them. A lady doctor from Allahabad says, 'I do not see the need for women doctors here, because male doctors are able to manage everything'. Look at the contradiction. Regarding puberty she says that in India it starts at the age of 9 or even before!

I think that I would give more accurate information on this subject. The Americans, I think, imagine anything, no matter what the reality may be. One of the foolish questions asked by the woman doctor was, 'Does India have many women?' She said, 'I hear that it is your custom to kill a baby girl as soon as she is born! This country [America] has more women than men, but there must be relatively few women in India if female infants are killed'. This is the wisdom and progress of the Westerners whom we praise so much! And so, if they imagine us to be the middle link between monkeys and humans, it would not be surprising! What a dreadful idea! I did not know that India is such a barbaric and cruel country! Also, until I met these people, I did not know that India is so heathen. They think that everything cruel and barbaric happens only in heathen countries. One hears these ideas everywhere. You can imagine how it pains me. I feel no shame if they use the word in its literal sense. I would say that I too am an unbeliever. And I am proud of it. (That is the difference between myself and others.) I am very proud of being a Hindu. After a while I said, 'But I do not believe this. At least in the nineteenth century, there is no such thing in India. Would it not be better to discuss this with some knowledgeable people before you speak?' I cannot imagine that they are so ill-informed. I am not exaggerating or making up an amusing story; nor is this idle talk. I am saying this not rashly, but after careful and proper consideration. There is no room for doubt. Women in America and England have all facilities. They are believed to be superior to other women in the whole world. Besides, thousands of people from these countries go to India every year. So naturally they are more knowledgeable. Is it better to spend more brains on such wild conjectures and foolish questions – which are as difficult to understand as to answer! We Indian women who are without status, deprived of our rights by men, and more backward in every way, are still better than them! It is worth remembering that being inherently weak, we have had to cultivate the typically Indian fortitude in order to protect morality, religion and intellect! Every nation should emulate Indian women and learn endurance from them. They may be superstitious, ignorant, misguided, or may hold wrong beliefs, but [they] can hardly be blamed. Since all laws, rules, customs, etc., are favourable to men, it is not surprising or improbable that the women have remained in this state. I do not like to harp on the past; but unless the past and present are compared, the future cannot be predicted. We must understand how we have reached this state. We must see what is wrong with the past and present women. We must also understand why, when and how men respected us or protected us from enemies, or deprived us of our rights. Instead of grieving about the present, or resenting the good fortune of others, one should concentrate on how to escape from ignorance. One must remember that the future is still to come and has not yet passed. Please note how often I have to beg your pardon so that you do not misunderstand me . . .

Your letter of the 29*th* [January] criticising Doctor Thoburn has just arrived. I do not repent that the truth is out. . . . But I only hope that my readers respect my truthfulness. Meaning is often distorted and exaggerations are common. That is why I requested you not to show my letters to anybody else. Besides, there is nothing in them worth showing. I am sorry that you disregard my wish. It is sad that we do not share the same views these days. You say that you despise Indians. You hold them in contempt and are impatient to voice your opinion. I really do not understand why. I never hate any people or religion. I have no enemy, and I think I never will. I feel the same love towards all. . . . I think that is obstinacy [on your part] and do not like it. I pity such narrow-mindedness. Should I defend your faults, mischief and hypocrisy, just because they are yours? . . .

You told me to describe everything I see before me, but I have been unable to do so because I am afraid of creating the wrong impression (by describing a person or his behaviour as I see it). There is a new fashion of wearing girdles. Already the practice of tight-lacing makes it impossible to breathe freely, and now this fashion! This is the way to improve upon progress! If the Chinese bind their feet, it is because they are ignorant and idolators. If Westerners do such things, it is because they are very advanced! Happy are the women who are free from such foolish things!

I think that the women here are much more prone to gynaecological disorders than the simple and wise Indian women. I would rather remain ignorant than become a Christian. There is an opposition between this culture and improved health care. These women are justly punished for their stupidity and empty conceit. Being all alone among them, I fear being persuaded, but pray that this will not happen.

. . . I feel very sorry that Rao Saheb Dandekar tried to prejudice you against me. . . . [It] is not fitting that an elderly and wise man should do so against one whom he considers to be like his own daughter, and that makes me sad!

Please do not think that I would prevent you from doing anything good, but I will always give you my opinion.

The news that the Ilbert Bill has passed has overjoyed me. Indeed we should thank God and be ever grateful to this true friend of the Indian people!

My papers in the Preliminary Examination have gone well. . . . Now I work in the College. Today is Monday, and I have been standing for about five hours at a stretch and am feeling very tired. Since my last illness, I start trembling as soon as I get tired. I had gone to visit Aunt, and spent the time happily. After finishing this, I am going to write a letter to my mother. I was not able to study for some time, so I was afraid that I might lose a whole year. I did not stand first in the examination, but I think I will in the final examination next year. . . . my health is all right. I feel unwell if I do not work at all. But I will take care not to exert myself too much.[9]

*

The Joshees' marital storms were usually provoked by Gopalrao's increasingly frequent and bitter complaints about Anandibai's tardy letters and allegedly conceited and Westernised ways. His frustration at his own stagnation while she was exploring a new country and culture, and enjoying the limelight, was palpable. It was almost a repetition of his childhood feelings of insecurity and inferiority when confronted by his smartly turned out, English-speaking Mumbai friend. Particularly acrimonious was his latest diatribe about Anandibai's change of costume, allegedly without his prior permission. His wrath was further fuelled by a photograph she had sent him, in which her shoulders and bust were not modestly covered as they should have been. A resigned Anandibai replied in early [March?] 1884:

Your letter of 6th January 1884 is just at hand. If there is anything left in our unfortunate India which gives you satisfaction, I beg of you to inform me of it, for I am unable to see it. Even as your faithful wife, I can do nothing to please you. Since the Merciful God has given me a human life and sent me into this world, I accept it with great humility, equanimity and loyalty. He knows what is good or bad for his poor hapless children.

You have criticised my dress with heavy sarcasm. In fact, you had anticipated a change in my costume, but I had not anticipated such severe criticism of it. I am astonished that people forget so easily what they have said or written. I clearly remember your advice to me to dress like Englishwomen, if necessary. You wrote to Mrs Carpenter and also to me that I should even eat meat, if necessary. Now I don't know whether you did so only to test my resolve. But I do only what I think right and have not followed your advice. I have not done so even after you told me to. I admit my mistake in not informing you immediately of the change I made in my dress. But there was hardly any time to obtain your consent, because the sudden change of weather on the steamer compelled me to make certain alterations in my dress, and I did what was right according to my conscience. I had only my conscience to advise me. In your letter you have criticised the blouse I wore in the photograph, but I promise you I never thought of it. I am sorry it made you unhappy. The *padar* of the *pitambar* fell off my shoulder not because of carelessness, but inadvertently. I was not aware of it, nor was anybody else. That is why the photograph was taken as it was. I know only too well that the fault will be mine, if I do anything to incur public censure. Usually I do not act without proper consideration. I think it better to cut off the organ which is likely to harm the whole body. I wear my current dress only for protecting my health. This Gujarati dress is a part of our country, and therefore I do not find it improper in any way, nor is there any flippancy or showing off. I like the Maharashtrian style of sari and blouse, and I know that you want me to continue with it. You also know of my resolve to do so. But the circumstances are quite unfavourable. I have no tears left to pay the penalty for having given you so much pain. I am not even able to heave a sigh. I only have a 'heart' which melts or freezes at your warm or cold words. I feel sorry not for myself, but because I am unable to give you happiness or satisfaction. I tell you this from the bottom of my heart. . . .

It is not at all my intention to distress you dear heart or to cause a rift in our love by raking up old memories. I only beg you to cultivate patience. Don't misunderstand me and make me suffer so. It is very difficult to decide whether your treatment of me was good or bad. If you ask me, I would answer that it was both. It seems to have been right in view of its ultimate goal; but, in all fairness, one is compelled to admit that it was wrong, considering its possible effects on a child' mind. Hitting me with broken pieces of wood at the tender age of ten, flinging chairs and books at me and threatening to leave me when I was twelve, and inflicting other strange punishments on me when I was fourteen – all these were too severe for the age, body, and mind at each respective stage. In childhood the mind is immature and the body undeveloped. And you know how I acted on these occasions. If I had left you at that immature age, as you kept on suggesting, what would have happened? I would have been lost. (And any number of girls have left their homes because of harassment from mothers-in-law and husbands.) I did not do so because I was afraid that my ill-considered behaviour would tarnish my father's honour. . . . And I begged you not to spare me, but to kill me. In our society, for centuries there has been no legal restraint between husbands and wives; and if it exists, it works against women! Such being the case, I had no recourse but to allow you to hit me with chairs and bear it with equanimity. A Hindu woman has no right to utter a word or to advise her husband. On the contrary, she has a right to allow her husband to do what he wishes and to keep quiet. Every Hindu husband can, with advantage, learn patience from his wife. (I do understand that without you I would never have become what I am now, and I am eternally grateful to you; but you cannot deny that I was always calm.) I was born to endure all that. But I am quite content now.

My mother too never spoke to me affectionately. When she punished me, she was wont to use not just a small rope or thong, but always stones, sticks and live charcoal. Fortunately, my body does not bear any scars, and her severe beatings did not leave me maimed, crippled or deformed. By the grace of God, my limbs survived intact! But oh! the sheer agony of those memories! But this has not diminished my love for my mother after the passage of childhood. Truly, she never understood the duties of a mother, nor did I experience the love which a child naturally feels for its mother. This memory hurts me a great deal. A child which harbours fear for its parents cannot possibly feel affection for them, and a child which feels love for its parents does not fear them. Unfortunate indeed is the child which has missed a happy childhood. I feel perfectly certain that, having understood the problem, I would be able to solve it. If I ever have a child, I will teach people by my own example how children should be brought up.[10]

This letter, clear-sightedly outlining Gopalrao's aggressive and even violent treatment of her since early childhood, juxtaposed with Anandibai's deep and oft-expressed love for him, brings out all the contradictions in this complex marital relationship. Her independent spirit and professed dependence on him is part of the contradiction, as is her shifting awareness of a separate identity and submergence in his. In an earlier letter to Gopalrao, perhaps in 1883, Anandibai had written

> I cannot tell you how eager I am to meet you. Your letters are very sweet. They provide me the only solace I have. I don't know what would have happened to me without them. That is why I am grateful to the person who discovered the art of letter-writing. Only your last letter is somewhat strange. It shows that you are troubled and uneasy about something; I wish you had told me what. I wish to be near you to comfort you when you are uneasy. . . . Just as you share your happiness with me, share your sorrows also. So far, nobody knows my mind except you. But even you will never fathom its depth.[11]

Probably in the spring of 1884, Anandibai wrote to Gopalrao about her ideas on the evolution of the species, and how the nineteenth-century Western science had only proved what the ancient Hindu sacred books had already outlined through the ten incarnations of Vishnu.

*

During the same spring, Anandibai encountered insane patients in the College and in the Morristown Insane Asylum. She shared these unimagined adventures with either Gopalrao or Mrs Carpenter:

> I met a mad woman for the first time in the College Hospital. One day our professor demonstrated the post-mortem dissection which was performed by a woman in the senior class, in which I assisted. When everything was over, the professor and students left the operating room and I was standing alone by the dissection table. Mrs Smith was putting on her hat on the terrace. Just then, a mad woman rushed in, uttering a terrible sound, and saw me standing by the table in which lay the dissected body with the heart and other organs beside it, and surrounded by surgical instruments. Seeing that nobody else was around, she seemed to harbour some suspicion in her insane mind. With a cruel expression on her face, she demanded to know why I had come there and what I was doing. I did not

answer her and I did not even stir. From her general demeanour, I had already guessed that she was quite insane. She seemed to be stronger than I, and capable of using the instruments lying there if she wanted to. But she was obviously afraid of me. I did not move from that spot, because I thought she would follow me, but I was not in the least afraid of her. She kept on firing questions at me. I did not reply to any. I thought that if I spoke, it would trigger off a fit of insanity in her. Mrs Smith was frightened when she saw her, knowing better than I what type of a person she was. She signalled to me to escape and save myself. At last, when I was withdrawing little by little, her attendant came in search of her and took her away.[12]

A somewhat less eventful visit to the Asylum followed shortly, when 'an insane woman rushed forward to shake my hand and another hugged me so tightly that I could free myself only by distracting her with a long conversation'. Yet another woman threw a pillow at her as she was about to leave the ward, and a group of male inmates suddenly accosted her and blocked her path.[13]

*

A revealing and somewhat intriguing event occurred in the spring of 1884: Anandibai gave an address before a ladies' missionary society on the subject of 'Early Marriage' which was reported to Gopalrao on 3 May 1884:

> Your letter arrived; I was overjoyed. The Sanskrit books have arrived, for which I thank you. I am exhausted because of the overload of work, but not ill.
>
> At the missionary meeting, there was a debate of 'Child Marriage'. About two thousand women had assembled, some had to turn back for want of room. I had not had time to write a single word of my speech due to work, and spoke extempore. I got an award of 10 dollars. During the vacation I have to study. If I get time, I will prepare, that is write out, another lecture on the topic 'Hindu Women'. Balji's book has come, but will not be at all useful for my lectures. They will be based on my own thoughts and experiences. Never mind. I receive several invitations to lecture, but I always refuse them and will continue to do so. Because I can only do what is possible after managing my studies.

I cannot describe the happiness I felt because you have started a good deed on our New Year's Day [Gudi Padwa]. Instead of opening a poor asylum, it would be far better to start a school for orphans. I will help you in this project when I return. There are many poor asylums, but not enough schools for orphans. If I am told to give my life for the orphans of India, I would not feel sad. I pray to God that you will make a similar resolution.[14]

Anandibai's talk in support of child marriage, so cursorily mentioned, stunned and embarrassed her progressive friends. They tried to explain it away in their own ways. Dr Bodley traced her conservative views to strongly internalised (though ultimately detrimental) norms, it being 'absolutely impossible' for 'a high-caste Hindu wife to speak otherwise'. She also discovered 'in the herculean attempt of that occasion, a clue to the influences which at length overpowered and slew this gentle, grave woman'.[15] Mrs Dall saw it as an expression of Anandibai's own positive experience of child marriage, coupled with the negative image she might have formed of the conjugal disharmony in America:

I think it tried the patience of those who were interested in her very severely. I have never seen any abstract of her remarks, but if she favored early marriages, was it strange? She had been married at nine years. All the happiness of her life had flowed from the instruction of her husband, and from that liberal sympathy which she supposed to move him in assisting her to come to this country. When she arrived, she found our papers full of conjugal quarrels, and applications for divorce. Not in one year nor twenty could she be expected to solve the problems whose very existence filled her with disgust.[16]

There is no other record of this talk, nor is Anandibai's reasoning known. However, Gopalrao's defence of child marriage was published in a newspaper article about a year later, on his arrival in America. Anandibai's own earlier vacillation on the topic in her correspondence with Mrs Carpenter has already been described. On the whole this seems to have been a case partly of strongly interiorised patriarchal norms and partly of a nationalist defence of Indian customs she may have private reservations about – especially when confronted by the missionaries who so openly flaunted their Orientalist contempt for Indian customs.

*

Notes

1 Dall, p. 107.
2 Ibid, p. 108.
3 Kanitkar, p. 224, my translation.
4 Ibid, pp. 176–77, my translation.
5 Ibid, p. 215, my translation.
6 Ibid, pp. 197–98.
7 Ibid, p. 199.
8 Here Anandibai draws a triangle for the Christian Trinity and compares it with a Hindu Trinity of Brahma, Vishnu and Shiva.
9 Kanitkar, p. 209.
10 Ibid, p. 189, my translation.
11 Ibid, p. 195, my translation.
12 Ibid, p. 233, my translation.
13 Ibid, p. 234.
14 Ibid, p. 213, my translation.
15 Bodley, 'Introduction', pp. ii–iii.
16 Dall, p. 109.

11

A FAMILY REUNION

When the *Mahratta* (22 June 1885) sympathetically suggested that Anandibai 'must be sadly in want of a companion' and that 'her husband . . . should join her soon', she herself had been literally counting the days until their next meeting:

> Today it is exactly one year, two months and twenty days since you and I parted. This separation is becoming intolerable. I try to immerse myself in work at all times to avoid being overcome by despondency. It is better for the mind to be diverted with books or some other thoughts. Will these dry letters be able to express my love for you? They will not have that power unless they are read with eyes equally full of love. You will not be able to imagine my condition – how can you, when I myself am unable to describe it? I feel that my heart is swaying like a boat; but my real heart is very far away, with you. No matter what the distance, it will not be separated from you, ever. This being the case, why talk of separation at all? But one must, because my physical self is far away from you . . .
>
> Do you feel any concern for me at all? . . . I had been hoping that you would arrive soon. But 'man proposes and God disposes'. . . . I would be happier in a dark cell with you, than alone in a palace![1]

The letter (presumably dated 27 June 1884) found Gopalrao somewhere on his travels to the United States via Burma, China, and Japan.

*

For over a year Gopalrao had chafed at his stagnant routine in Bengal and longed to share with his wife her – and his own – adventures. His departure was precipitated by an incident when his superior in the postal department pulled him up for no fault of his own. The gravely offended Gopalrao resigned from his job in a fit of temper (without informing Anandibai, who found this out much later) and despite the kindly Mr James' intercession on his behalf, Anandibai was to allude to the event in a letter to her brother-in-law in January 1886:

> He knew whether he was doing right or wrong. . . . [I]f Mr James had not advised my husband the way he did (and that itself was an excellent test of his friendship), I would not have respected him as a friend. But Mr James proved his true and sincere friendship. Now, whether Mr Joshee behaved accordingly is another question.[2]

Gopalrao was now freed from financial responsibility for Anandibai by the generous 'James Fund'. Mr James's circular mentioned that 'a young Brahmin lady had gone to America recently' to qualify as a medical doctor to help 'native ladies', having made 'pecuniary sacrifices'. He wanted to raise a fund 'in recognition of her courage and public spirit' so that her tuition fees could be covered. He himself subscribed Rs 200, and all the high British officials from the viceroy and the governor-general to the chief justice of Calcutta High Court contributed various sums so that Rs 750 were collected and conveyed to Anandibai.[3]

In mid-June 1884, Gopalrao embarked on his liberating adventure – 'in search of truth and a land where my heart will be at rest', as the *Mahratta* (13 July 1884) reported. The journey took him eastward to explore India's immediate neighbours in preference to the usual western route traversed by all other travellers (and most recently by his own wife) – perhaps to assert his distinctiveness, or perhaps as the first leg of his projected journey around the world. At any rate, the unusual pan-Asian solidarity which infused his travel accounts provides a glimpse of his bold and original thinking as much as his practical sense, which foresaw India's increased Asian trade connections.

In the true spirit of adventure, Gopalrao had booked himself as a deck passenger 'to save money and secondly to see how poor people are taken care of on board the steamer'. This decision he regretted soon enough, admitting that 'my voyage was neither cheap nor comfortable; on the contrary I . . . suffered so much that my life was at stake'. After landing at Rangoon (now Yangon) on 22 June, he discovered further risks. Forced to take shelter in a temple and disappointed in his search for free food allegedly distributed by a generous Indian, he finally ended his starvation of four days by getting 'one Madrasi Brahmin family to cook for me, at my own expense'. However, he was enterprising enough to have this account of his voyage published in the *Rangoon Gazette* of 26 June 1884, with an editorial written about it, and to have the *Mahratta* (13 July 1884) publish both under the ambitious rubric 'Some account of Burmah'.

Rangoon impressed him greatly by its 'beautiful scenery' which 'refreshes everything both physical and mental', in contrast to Mumbai, Calcutta, and Madras. The city was 'systematically laid out' and clean, with good sanitary arrangements which did much credit to the English. But more impressive were the people, largely engaged in trade, who refused to serve others: 'Not a Burman [sic] to be found to carry your loads, to sweep your ground, to cook for you, or to beg alms for you'. This national pride prevented them from kowtowing to the British, so that 'No Englishman can speak ill of the Burman with impunity just as he does in India'. Equally impressive was the discovery that the Buddhist Burmese felt an affinity with Hindu Indians as brothers in religion – while narrow-minded Indians would not reciprocate the sentiment.

The next instalment of the travelogue in the *Mahratta* (2 November 1884) was 'An Account of Siam' – 'a fertile valley whose wealth is beyond calculation', although each inhabitant from the king down to the peasant 'is still savage in appearance'. Gopalrao invited young enterprising Indians to seek better contacts with Southeast and East Asia. He continued via Saigon, Annam, and Tonquin to China which, in his opinion, was another country worth exploring by Indian enterprise, contrary to the popular perception in India (a point he made through some name-dropping). As for the Chinese, 'there has not been a nobler, more patriotic and more loving and peaceful race created by God than the Chinese'. Direct interaction with them would bring India reciprocal benefits.

Struck by this novel pan-Asian vision – an unusual extension of nationalism which questioned India's Western orientation and perception of its neighbours only through Western eyes – the *Mahratta* highlighted it in an editorial note in the same issue.

Both Joshees were now squarely in the limelight as the chosen figureheads for the newly educated, socio-politically conservative Maharashtrians represented by the *Kesari-Mahratta* group. Their path-breaking travels, innovative ideas, and new ventures served well as a weapon to target both the social reformers – 'pseudo-reformers who only 'preached' but did not 'practise' their radical ideas as the Joshees were now doing – and Pandita Ramabai, a 'religious zealot' who was already in England and doing well, but whose nationalist credentials were suspect because of her conversion.

*

In March 1884, Anandibai passed the first-year examination, an event which did not go unreported in Maharashtra. Both the *Mahratta* and *Kesari* seized the opportunity to compare Anandibai favourably with Pandita Ramabai, who had recently been appointed Professor of Sanskrit and the Vernacular Languages at the Cheltenham Ladies' College.[4] The *Mahratta* adopted a liberal tone, but *Kesari* vented its full antagonism against Ramabai while adding a warm personal note about Anandibai, and singling out Gopalrao for special credit.

*

During the summer vacation that followed, Anandibai visited Mrs Carpenter's cousin Mrs Barto at Saratoga, famous for its natural springs and salubrious climate. Her enjoyment was marred by ill health, though she tried to make light of it in her letter to Mrs Carpenter:

> Ever since I left Roselle, I have not spent a day without my new companion, the headache. Every moment gives me pain, but you need not worry about it, because I do not let it interfere with anybody's happiness, nor even with my own. One day at Troy we had cucumber pickles; the pickles looked unnaturally green. I suspected copper in them, so I took a needle and ran it into one of the cucumbers. In a few minutes I was satisfied, for the needle had turned bright red.[5]

At about this time Anandibai also visited a number of educational institutions.[6] But she did not enjoy Barnum's Circus, confessing to Mrs Carpenter: 'Such places bore and disgust me. But Miss B kept on inviting me for more than a month, so I felt obliged to go'.[7]

All too soon it was time to return to college and its hectic schedule. Anandibai wrote from Philadelphia on 9 October to Mrs Carpenter:

> Excuse me for not writing earlier. College opened on Thursday, October *2nd*; the opening address was by Professor Parish; it was a charming lecture, useful and interesting to every individual, the subject being Practical Hygiene. It was timely, and benefitted me as well as the general public. He had a large audience. The day after, work began; I have to attend all the lectures except those on Materia Medica and Surgery, which I take up next year. I work from fifteen to sixteen hours daily. The day after College began, Mrs Smith and I went to the Electrical Exhibition in the evening and enjoyed it very much. I enjoy my studies more than ever. Professor Wite [?] came only three

days ago, so we had our first lecture on Physics yesterday. I am grieved to tell you I am to lose an excellent friend and teacher. The sickness of Dr Emily Du Bois, Demonstrator of Anatomy, was sudden to us all; but *she knew it before*. Faithful, prompt and thorough, she neglected her own self.

I have not taken money on the cheque just received from the James fund. As I had enough trouble in trying to have another cashed, on account of the wrong spelling of my name ['Joshi' instead of 'Joshee'?], I did not try to borrow any more trouble that day. I have so little time to spare. I have not a cent with me, but owe a little to Mrs Smith, and cannot get to clinics for the same reason. I have had a severe cold for a week, and am aching all over.[8]

In her letter to Bapusaheb Ketkar on 8 October, Anandibai mentioned that she had seen her first surgical operation recently, and one of the new students fainted. She herself had registered her name for post-mortem dissection and awaited her turn.[9] Soon afterwards she wrote to Ketkar, urging him to trace her horoscope and send it to her urgently, along with a Hindu calendar of the year of her birth, so that she could check something very important.[10]

*

In November 1884 Govindrao Sathe arrived from Calcutta and visited Anandibai at Roselle, carrying many gifts (saris and 'embroidered jackets') for Anandibai and the Carpenters. He was the first Maharashtrian she had conversed with since her unfortunate meetings with Rajwade and Guruji a year earlier, and the Carpenters found it 'delightful to hear the cadences of the Mahratta tongue once more'.[11]

Anandibai paid her first visit to Mrs Dall in her Georgetown house in Washington D.C. in December 1884. The train was late and the carriage engaged by Dall had gone by the time she arrived.

We were obliged to go out in a horse-car, and this was not desirable on account of the attention she could not fail to attract. Beside this, she had some heavy hand baggage which she would not let me carry up the hill. I remember with surprise the calmness with which she endured the curious gaze of our companion, and the courage with which she bore her burden and encountered the necessary fatigue. She was a striking contrast to the English ladies who came over to Philadelphia with the British Association that same year. During her stay with me I took her to all the public buildings, to a service at the Unitarian church, to several private lunches, to dine with Commodore Walker's family and two other friends, and to several receptions. Nowhere did any peculiar awkwardness draw any attention to her foreign education.

It pleased her to draw quietly about my house, taking up and touching the various articles that had been sent from India.[12]

The attention Anandibai attracted was considerable, as Mrs Dall noted in her diary on 29 December 1884:

A very unpleasant day, but we had fifty-two callers, and in the evening gave a light supper to thirty. Last evening Mrs Joshee talked well about the antiquity of her nation, and of her family record, which she asserts is two thousand years old. She promises to write me details about it, and to lend me some of the peculiar paper upon which it is written, when she returns home. Tonight, before quite a large company, she talked in an earnest and excited way about the religions of the world, showing a profound intelligence as well as scholarship. Then for a while in a very entertaining way about jewels and costumes. Her best talk was with the Rev. Theodore Winkoop, after most of our friends had gone.

Tonight she wore a close satin vest embroidered with gold, and a white camel's hair shawl or saree [?] deeply bordered with gold; also her collars and necklaces of jewels, and for the first time, at my request, her 'nose-ring'. This is a spray of flowers, two or three inches long, and made of fine old pearls. The pearls were some of those given by the king to her warlike ancestor in Poonah. The centers of the starlike flowers are of ruby and emerald. A fine wire attaches it to the left nostril close to the cheek. It is very effective, much prettier than ear-rings, and looks as if she were holding a spray of flowers between her lips.[13]

Dall's account shows either a communication gap or an unwarranted exaggeration on Anandibai's part. A family history going back two thousand years is clearly impossible, as is a camel-hair sari. The American fascination with nose-rings has also been noticed in Mrs Carpenter's case.

*

Gopalrao finally arrived in the United States in the spring of 1885, landing at California, and immediately made waves through the American newspapers. The excited Anandibai was confronted by fresh dilemmas. The seemingly minor question of the greeting appropriate for their first meeting acquired major proportions in view of her surreptitious acculturation over the previous two years. She broached the subject to him, along with other news, on 13 March 1885:

> I have passed all the examinations this year. I am sure this news will please you too. God willing, I will get my degree next year. I am hopeful. I have been too busy the last fortnight to write to you.
>
> As the time of our meeting draws near, let us talk about ourselves. Who can fathom the joy I feel at the thought of the near future? But this kind of happiness is always fraught with obstacles. Let us give some though as to where, how and when we are to meet in June, and what our next step should be. In June I will go to Roselle, and I beg you to come there first. Where should we meet? I think we will all come to New York to receive you, and then we will stay at home in Roselle for a few days. Now I request your instructions with regard to the manner of our meeting. When a distant male relative (like a cousin or a second cousin) arrives, women kiss him at their first meeting. Men do not kiss each other, but they kiss a sister, mother, wife or daughter. If I do not kiss my dear husband on meeting him after a prolonged absence, my friends and those present will surely be scandalised. However, if an Indian woman kisses her husband in public, our people will think her shameless. I want to check this with you in advance because you are very particular about these things, and that there should be no confusion or doubt.
>
> Prof. Bodley had approached you through me regarding a job. I can vouch for your being an excellent teacher, but to accept the job of teaching Sanskrit without prior preparation will be foolhardy in my opinion. Teaching means an invitation to public scrutiny and criticism. Besides, even that job is not guaranteed. All colleges already have their own teachers and do not seem to need more. In this situation we must find an alternative ourselves. The one which has occurred to me is to earn money by giving lectures. I can see that this sounds like a clumsy suggestion, but it is the best by far. I am not too proud or greedy, but I too have ambition. We should think these things through while it is still in our hands. It would be best if we go hand in hand as usual.

One should think carefully before making a promise, and tell the truth. I am so preoccupied with important matters that diverting my mind to other things imposes an additional burden on me. If I need money, it is not for personal ornamentation, but for my studies which are dear to me. Without money I can do nothing. I need it at every step. One should either have money to one's heart's content, or be prepared for total disappointment. What have I learnt so far, and how much knowledge have I acquired, that I should lose interest in studies?

Since I have the means now, let me taste the nectar of knowledge to the full. Perhaps tomorrow my situation will change altogether, and I will be removed from the treasure of knowledge and the means of acquiring it. We can think further about this when we meet, just now I have only touched upon the matter in passing. I beg you to think about it and write to me accordingly. The people here are quite ignorant about India, so it would be good if you give them authentic information.

There is something I must divulge to you and prepare you for. I am certain that it will amuse, surprise and also anger you. I cannot speak Marathi! It is truly my own fault; but I wished with all my heart to become proficient in English and medicine. I have not forgotten Marathi altogether. I will be able to write, speak and also understand it. But I have lost the habit of speaking Marathi during the last two years. I have concentrated on my studies at the cost of everything else. Although it is not possible that I will forget my mother-tongue, my concentration on the English language and constant use of it have made it my native tongue! Even so, I am certain that if I re-acquaint myself with my mother-tongue for twenty hours, it will come back to me. You know my temperament well. I immerse myself in whatever I am doing at the moment, and forget everything I was doing the minute before! If you speak to me in Marathi patiently when we are alone, you will do for me what I want. . . . Whenever I wish, I will be able to speak Marathi as before, with a little practice; but nobody seems to realise the need for this. I have scribbled this in the few minutes which were left. I have informed everybody in India about my results and had kept this to the last so as to have sufficient time to think of important things. I had no wish at all to write about this [manner of greeting at the first meeting], but was compelled to, because you do not say a word about it and the time has come.

I have a headache today. I think this is only the second time since October 1884. I really do not know what I have written and where I have digressed. But I am hoping to recover from all these illnesses as soon as your letter comes. My second letter will appear even stranger than the first; but I think that an illness is aggravated after going out, as it is after a meal. There is an interesting mixture of cold, rain, haze, etc., outside. I will not re-read this, because I will find it too poor to send. But although the letter is so bad, I remain,

Your dear wife Yamuna[14]

Gopalrao's reaction to the letter was violent, and was countered by Anandibai (in late March 1885) with a calm tolerance laced with sarcasm:

Your letter is at hand. I cannot describe the happiness I derived from it, nor will I attempt to. I only beg you to continue giving me the benefit of your advice. You call me irritable, but I am certain that you will soon stop saying so. Your criticism about the quality of my letter is well-deserved, but rest assured that except for those letters, you will find no other so poor and full of mistakes. . . . if you can imagine my work load, lack of time and the number of meaningless but regular letters I receive, you will pardon me for neglecting something I love. Surely you know how essential it is to answer such people's letters, although most of them are casual scribblers or missionaries. Aunt's and your own letters are my only source of pleasure apart from studies. Don't think for a minute that I saying this only to please you, because you know that I am not one to do such a thing. There is nothing at all in this world which can take your place. Am I not aware of what you have done for me on the strength of your words, and am I not grateful for it? You are my guide, master, comforter and saviour. Moreover, I will always be grateful because you have freed me from slavery and carried me to the highest status possible for a woman.

I was hurt by your words, 'I do not need your advice'. If such a thought ever enters my immature mind, I will consider myself the lowest of the low and the meanest of the mean! If I ever consider myself to be omniscient, that would be the end of me! One word from you appears to me like the calm after a storm! I only beg of you, let it never come to my ears that you now hesitate to advise me the way you did earlier. Let us speak candidly to each other in this manner and find out the truth.

I think I have written to you whatever I know about Govindrao. There is no letter from him since he left Roselle, and that is not my fault. My college will close on the 30*th* of this month, and then I will go to Roselle. You have not yet informed me of your plans and when you have decided to meet me.

Did you go to Salt Lake City? If you wish, I would suggest that you visit Warrensburg and Missouri. (They are 200 miles from St. Louis.) I have a friend there, named Frances Coleman Smith, MD You should meet her because she really wants you to. She told me when she left that she would write to you about staying with her. She is a very good woman and was here with me for two years. She got her degree on 1*st* March and returned to her husband. He is also an expert in Anatomy and an excellent man. If you are planning to go there, I will inform you accordingly in advance. She sincerely wants me also to spend a few days with her during the vacation, but I am afraid I have too many difficulties.

Your lecture on the topic, 'Good Women', has caused a lot of stir in this city and all around. Many of my friends here are angry. Those who know that you are a true friend of the female sex, assert that you would never speak so ill of women. Some say that this is a fabrication of the newspapers. Others say that you have repented having sent your wife here for further education! It seems that they implicitly believe whatever you have said. People derive a kind of pleasure from spreading false reports about other countries, and they are very happy to think that you have supported their views. What amazing folly! I do not at all feel sorry, because I am convinced that you would never say anything improper or without a good motive. Have you decided when you are to come to Roselle? After such a long separation, I must come there to meet you.

Now I don't know what to write, although there seemed to be so much when I started. But as thoughts of you crowded into my mind, I started to forget what to write. What I do in my dreams seems to me better than what I do when I am awake. When I start writing to you, my hand trembles and words fail me. Please let me know your plans immediately, and believe me to be ever

Your dear wife Yamuna.[15]

Anandibai's next letter was written on 30 March 1885, on the eve of her twentieth birthday:

I need not beg your pardon for the flutter I was in and the hasty letters I wrote, because you know what a wife's love for her husband is like, no matter how foolish! Your letter which had just arrived led me to assume, perhaps childishly so, that you need a good rest before starting out on your travels again. And I heard just a few days ago that your future plans are changed. In replying to your letter written immediately on landing in America, I have made a couple of suggestions. After a few days I also wrote that you should come straight to me before everything else. I beg you to keep in mind both my letters and recognise my motive before making your plans. Now you are here, and have the world before you. I know that you really are what people think you are. Many will be surprised at you. And more will even try to test you. Of course you know what to do on such occasions – whatever seems right to you. I can say no more. You will do whatever is wise and proper. I have been waiting for your letter; there hasn't been one for a long time.

I have not uttered a word anywhere about Govindrao, but I cannot help saying that I am severely disappointed at his indecision and lack of purpose. His own words reveal his fickleness. Perhaps I am unduly inquisitive, or have misunderstood matters, but even so, I do not think that I am distorting the truth. He himself has never divulged his plans to me. . . .

I am faced with a profound question as to whether the people of India are honest. Whether Mother India is unfit, or whether we ourselves are dishonest and disobedient, and which of these has caused her present sorry plight, remains to be proven. The thought that we are still asleep while our motherland is submerged in a sea of sorrows just freezes my heart. She is drowning, but who will stretch out a helping hand? It is not for us to desert her though many people would do so in adverse times and very few would be ready to save her. We should all remember what the Roman warrior said: 'It is better to say of a person that he should not have died than to say he should not have been born'. . . .

Did you meet Dr Brown? I am eager to know about your health and whether you are rid of your rheumatism yet. I am eager to know all this. Please let me know how you are doing and what you think of that place [California]. Please don't forget to get me some Californian marine plants if they can be easily procured. I long to have them in my collection, but they are not available elsewhere. I have never asked you for anything so far, so I need not think this is too much.

A card has come from Bhaskar, which I have kept for you to see. I have replied to him, to the effect that I will accept the position if it is guaranteed, but will not discuss the salary. I will let you, your friends, and the employers decide it and inform me. I too will give my considered opinion on the matter. These may not have been my exact words, but this was the gist. Let me have your reaction. We should wait and watch the [Final Examination] results. Let me know if you meet Dr Brown. You never mentioned your meeting with Dr Mary Fulton at Canton, China. I heard about it from her, not you.

Tomorrow I will complete 20 years. When is your birthday? Prof. Bodley said in passing yesterday that you are a true well-wisher of women. Now you can see for yourself how much people admire you! I feel very proud of you.[16]

Had Anandibai misjudged the change that the two intervening years had wrought in Gopalrao, or had she always attributed to him liberal motives not strictly warranted by his behaviour? Had love and gratitude, which she repeatedly professed for him, blinded her to his flaws? And yet she seems to have been clear-sighted about his eccentricities, aggression, and violent temper in her letters. As she oscillated between sculpting a separate and strong identity for herself and submerging her identity in his – as she saw it, but not as it really was – she had perhaps lost sight of some of its salient facets. And the two-year absence while Anandibai went from strength to strength and Gopalrao stagnated and contented himself with basking in her reflected glory through newspaper publicity, perhaps hardened Gopalrao's frustration into envy of her achievements.

Gopalrao's arrival on the east coast of America was preceded by newspaper publicity caused by the public talks he gave on topics related to India. In Dall's words, 'The first notice of his coming was received through California newspapers which were sent to his wife's dearest friends'.[17] He was reported to have given an address in San Francisco which was unfavourable to the higher education of women because 'it unfitted them for the domestic duties of wives and mothers', and having hinted that his having sent his wife to study medicine in Philadelphia was a mistake. Anandibai herself made light of this in her letter cited above, but Dall noticed a 'subtle change' in her. Anandibai's friends were troubled but refrained from broaching the topic; however, when Dall's housekeeper in Washington, D.C., demanded an explanation from him (in Dall's absence), Gopalrao said he had made the speech 'just for a little fun; I thought it would stir them up a little'.[18]

News of Gopalrao's public speeches had also reached Maharashtra, probably sent by himself. The *Mahratta* (21 June 1885) reported his arrival in the United States and added:

> in an American paper we read an account of the lecture he delivered to a moderately sized audience at Washington. Mr Joshi [sic] takes a very gloomy view of our present condition and denounces the present rule for the misery it has brought upon India. We are sorry we cannot agree. . . . While here, Mr Joshi had the shackles of service on his feet and [a] humble situation in life did not bring him in contact with large-hearted European gentlemen. Besides, his transfer from Bombay to Bengal placed him in that part of the country where Anglo-Indianism is perhaps the strongest, so that what impressions he derived were of the dark side of the picture and not bright. But notwithstanding this our opinion. Mr Joshi cannot be much blamed for what he said: while speaking he had before him the picture of civilised and independent America and it was therefore quite natural that he should have forgotten the little blessings that we enjoy here.

A certain degree of embarrassment and desire to distance themselves from Gopalrao's presumably immoderate speeches were evident among the editors of the *Mahratta*. Perhaps this was their first glimpse of his feet of clay.

*

The cultural gap which seemed to have grown between the couple was further widened by Anandibai's admission that she had forgotten Marathi, implying that she had, equally surreptitiously, submerged totally into the American way of life. Despite her assurance of this being a temporary and easily rectifiable state of affairs, it is surprising in view of her emphatic nationalism. Gopalrao reacted with predictable hostility, accusing her of having betrayed her country and culture – a reaction shared by Govindrao Sathe. A beleaguered Anandibai replied:

> Never did I imagine that you would accuse me of disloyalty. How difficult it is to endure such a charge! It is unfortunate indeed that you have misunderstood what I wrote in my letter of the 13*th*, because it was not at all my intention to say that

either I or you have changed these days. It is best that you keep me under your supervision and show me the right path when I go astray. I can assure you that you wife is still in the same state that she was in when she parted from you. Only her dress has changed a little and her surroundings have changed, which is good and proper but temporary. It is not necessary for me to write further about it, or to beg forgiveness. I speak the very same language which you always advised me to master. My present situation is very different from that in India, which should be no surprise to you. Each one of my friends watches me all the time here, as if to test my character. I have heard from a stranger that the missionaries have said this about me: 'Mrs Joshee is exactly the same today as she was when she landed. There is not an iota of change in her. What a shame on Christianity, should she return to her native country in this state!' these were the words of an Episcopalian minister. This will show you how, without my knowledge, people are watching all my actions. When I asked you how we greet each other at our first meeting here, my intention was only to avoid confusion and blame to myself. If you wish to shake hands like strangers, I am willing to do so. Or if you think it proper for me to hang back timidly like a Hindu woman, I will do exactly that, although I have not done so in my life. It is not our custom for the wife to say 'Namaskar' to her husband, so obviously I cannot do that. Or if you wish, I can say 'How are you? I am glad to meet you' and then be silent. Of all these alternatives, if you prefer that I should pretend to be a shy Hindu woman, I will quickly retire to my room as soon as you arrive. Please do not laugh at all this. I really do believe that if we decide on one of these alternatives in mutual agreement, it would be best for both of us. I also like your plan to arrive at night.

Do you believe that I have become more greedy about money than I was? Because that is what I suspect from your writing. Earlier you used to send me money so that I was free to pursue my studies, and had no need to ask for money. But now that avenue is closed and I am compelled to give the matter some thought. If my education is provided for as before, I would not need a cent. You had written earlier that I should not touch the James fund'. Even so, except for 400 dollars, the rest of the fund has been spent, and I have not 22 dollars in hand. The scholarship I was awarded is also exhausted. I am very careful about spending money. I owe Dr Bodley about 40 dollars for my board. After paying her, I will have managed my College expenses for the year. This Professor is not wealthy, her income is moderate; how then can she afford to feed me free of charge? My dear aunt has so far not accepted a single cent from me. Suppose she had expected payment, how would I have paid her? This is not India, as you seem to forget sometimes. Once I thought I should sell my necklace; but when I tried, I found that it would not fetch one tenth its value. This is a golden opportunity to acquire knowledge and I am eager to acquire as much of it as possible. But nobody teaches you without charging exactly what it costs, or even more. I have not bought a single instrument yet, because surgical instruments cost hundreds of dollars, which I don't have. I will bide my time, but even you will admit that I must have instruments before I start my practice.

Is it better to depend on others for help than to earn yourself and live frugally? Oh no! I don't think you will ever agree. It is just that you seem to think that education is not costly. But you are mistaken. Do not for a moment entertain the thought that I now spend more money than before. On the contrary, you will be surprised to know how little I spend on myself. It is not that my living expenses are high but that my education – which appears to be free of charge – and clothes which cost a lot of money. Now there is only one thing left, that is to cut short my studies. But how can you or I entertain such a thought even in jest? When you come here, we will go and stay at Roselle. But I think it best for you to pay for your board, because Mr Carpenter is not rich enough to bear your expenses. I am confiding this only in you, and you will naturally assess the overall situation from this. I have not uttered a word in this regard to either Aunt or her husband, because how would you be able to pay so much? Actually we would not be able to repay them for the help they have extended to us, even if we live to be 200!

You will surely bear all these things in mind. I feel grieved at your habit of misinterpreting things. I did not at all mean to, even wish to, say that you treat me badly. I had only written about the excessive criticism Govindrao made of my having forgotten Marathi. He thought I had lost all my nationalism and become useless, and so he gave up all hope for me! He declared me totally unfit to return to my country or even show my face there. I do not consider this kind of talk worth more than punching the air. Besides, all this criticism was quite uncalled for and undeserved. Am I likely to find it difficult to speak Marathi if I really try? I don't think so at all. That I was able to speak fluent and grammatical English within 24 hours of leaving India, is proof enough of my claim. If you remember how little English I spoke in India and how ignorant I was of the language, you will agree that 24 hours would be too long [for me to start speaking Marathi again] . . .

Oh no! Will you stay there until I get my degree? Pray don't do any such thing. Come here as soon as you possibly can.

I have travelled 314 miles today to examine hospital patients, and am feeling quite bothered. My [letter-writing] days have already been fixed, yet I have had to write this letter in between, so it contains many faults which I hope you will overlook. I go there [to the hospital] every week. In addition to the College classes and this visit, there is another lesson scheduled there. I think I have sent you the College schedule. I would like to make a suggestion. Whenever a foreigner arrives in this country, he is followed by some reporter or another. And you have undoubtedly met a number of them already. So do be very careful about giving your opinion on any subject, because those who are not Christian or Mormon are likely to cause trouble. Salt Lake City is on your way, so do visit it. It is a beautiful city well worth seeing. Do write a travelogue too. I don't remember which of your questions remain unanswered, so if you repeat them I can reply accordingly. Aunt, her husband and children send their regards. Everybody is eagerly awaiting your arrival. Prof. Bodley's regards.[19]

Money seems to have been a bone of contention. In spite of Anandibai's frugal habits, Gopalrao's cavalier attitude to money matters and to his own financial responsibilities made things difficult for her.

When Gopalrao finally arrived at Roselle, he characteristically did so without prior notice. Anandibai had gone with Eighmie to visit friends and returned an hour after his arrival. When she entered the drawing room as usual, she saw him sitting by the table at the centre, reading.[20] The manner of their much-discussed first greeting remains unrecorded.

*

The effect of Gopalrao's arrival on Anandibai was difficult to assess. For one thing she had not imagined that instead of taking a few months' leave, he would resign his post. His arrival in the United States without any financial resources whatsoever added to her embarrassment. Mrs Dall comments that when she asked her why he had done so, she said briefly and with a deep sigh, 'He is tired', but would not pursue the subject. After his coming, he shared the generous and provident kindness which had been extended to her, but he received it differently, and she knew it.

This year presented peculiar causes for anxiety, and for Mr Joshee's excitability, dissatisfaction, and restlessness there is an excuse to be found in the condition of his wife's health, and the impossibility of tempting her appetite with suitable food wherever she might be. Gopal had entered the United States by the wrong gate. The restless life of the West, the disorganization of the border, did not give him the key he needed to understand the eastern states. He saw very little, but thought he saw everything. This, however, he did perceive, that Anandabai's health was failing, and unable to aid her himself, half-frantic with affection and anxiety, he required of us all what it was impossible to give. Little did he know that it was chiefly owing to Dr Bodley's tender foresight that his wife was still living. To provide her with an abundance of nutritious vegetable food was often impossible, and there was not a physician anywhere who would not have said she needed broth and delicate meats; but these she could not take.[21]

Mrs Dall herself was convinced that Gopalrao would 'make life impossible for her', and noticed a marked difference in her:[22]

> Whoever had walked the streets of Philadelphia in modest peace with Anandabai [sic], could not fail to find a difference when Gopal was added to the party. His excited manner, his loud and rapid talk attracted the attention of the crowd, and this was held by the floating blue wrap, the white scarf, and dark turban which he always wore.[23]

During the next four months, Gopalrao remained at Roselle with Anandibai, to recover his strength after the prolonged travels. He had ample opportunity to explore his surroundings in the Carpenters' company. Their excursions took them to New York City, where they attended the Sunday church services by Talmage and Ward Beecher at Brooklyn: Both of them expressed a wish to meet Anandibai and had a discussion with her. They also visited the Greenwood Country cemetery; Anandibai thought its beauty made it appropriate for those who had departed for the next world.[24] After four months, Anandibai and Gopalrao left for Philadelphia before college opened, in order to attend a friend's wedding, and also saw the sights, including the Swedish Church, said to be the oldest in America. Gopalrao then went alone to Washington, D.C., as Anandibai started her classes.[25]

Notes

1 Kanitkar, pp. 236, my translation.
2 Ibid, p. 81.
3 Dall, p. 113.
4 This professorship was somewhat misleading. Ramabai was studying to be a teacher at the College (in fact a girls' school with a teacher-training department), and was to teach any students desirous of working in India.
5 Dall, p. 111.
6 Ibid, p. 109.
7 Kanitkar, pp. 233, my translation.
8 Dall, pp. 111–12.
9 Kanitkar, pp. 211.
10 Ibid, pp. 212.
11 Dall, p. 114.
12 Ibid, pp. 117–18.
13 Ibid, p. 119.
14 Kanitkar, pp. 241–43, my translation.
15 Ibid, pp. 244–45, my translation.
16 Ibid, pp. 247, my translation.
17 Dall, p. 123.
18 Ibid, p. 124.
19 Kanitkar, pp. 251, my translation.
20 Ibid, p. 252.
21 Dall, pp. 137–39.
22 Ibid, p. 138.
23 Dall, p. 140. Mr William Cobb's collection of Anandibai's stuff includes a purplish blue stitched and stiff 'pagdi' as worn by Maharashtrian Brahmins, except that their usual colour was red. This was the only blue pagdi I have seen. Incidentally, it was too small for my head, suggesting that Gopalrao was rather short and had a spare bone structure.
24 Dall, p. 124; Kanitkar, p. 253.
25 Kanitkar, p. 253.

12

COMPLETING COLLEGE

In October 1885 Anandibai entered the final year of her medical course. After the first term was over, she spent her Christmas holidays with the Carpenters as usual, from 23 December 1885 to 4 January 1886.[1]

Probably Anandibai's very first letter of 1886 was written on 2 January to her husband's brother in India, and dwelt on her favourite theme, nationalism and social obligation. This brother-in-law (probably Bhaskar) had requested her to put in a word with Mr James (fearing that he had been alienated by Gopalrao's earlier capricious behaviour) to give him a position in the postal department, and possibly unwittingly incurred Anandibai's nationalistic wrath for his lack of spirit.

> I have now enjoyed a rest from the toil and exertion of my college work, although it has been a labour of love, and am able to give my free time to the long neglected housework. So, during these Christmas holidays, I am trying to complete all the unfinished chores. From the beginning of the letter you will see that I am once again visiting Aunt during the holidays. As you know, my husband has come here. And so the last year passed away happily. It affected me just like the spring blossoms which erase the depression of winter and gladden all creatures! You will probably not be able to share my experience because you have not seen such a severe winter. . . . my college course is also nearing completion, and I hope that my goal of obtaining the longed for degree will be achieved next March.
>
> I was planning to write this for a long time, but did not find the time because of the magnitude of work. It seems that you have given up your old plan, and the ambition to enter government service has now taken complete possession of your mind. Looking at it from your point of view, I cannot help feeling sad at this change of heart. Even considering it from

mine, I feel sad. Because, out of the few friends who share my ideas, one has given up his plan which had all the chances of success and thus lost the freedom of speech and action which very few people enjoy. I may be wrong, but the thing is that among the three of us (I, my husband and yourself), I have the widest experience of this world. Probably that is why I cannot understand what satisfaction you derive from your present plan. I am writing this letter in order to offer some suggestions as your well-wishing sister-in-law. Please do not misunderstand me. I am writing exactly what I would have told you, had you asked me. You may be sure that I would not wish to advise you. I do not at all consider myself your superior in age or wisdom; so the question of advising you does not arise. Have you forgotten your wise thoughts and words when we were together? Where are the happy thoughts of freedom in the heart bleeding for the motherland? Is it at all possible that they can have disappeared with the passage of time?

I was also tempted to make the same mistake when an excellent opportunity came my way through Mr James's kindness, but fortunately I was inspired by other thoughts which changed the direction of my life altogether. There was a time when I had humbled myself before others for a job in the Post Office. I was kindly offered a good job, suitable for my qualifications, at Rs 30 a month. But when the time came to give a definite answer, I was loath to sell my freedom for this job or even one offering five times the salary. Now I have only one regret. My example would have helped many other women, and those who are now struggling to get jobs would have been able to do so. This did not happen. I am just one among many other backward women. But even though I wanted a job, I never wanted to be like other people competing for petty jobs. So I found a small vocation which would help my country and other poor women like myself. You, my friend, are young and learned, and prepared to do anything for yourself. Such educated and courageous young men are rare to find, and when the time comes it is at their hands that India will be emancipated from her fallen state and will prosper. Foreigners have started hundreds of trades only for the natives who are prepared to take risks. When there are more jobs than workers, why do you complain? Don't you even think of an art, craft, trade or profession which would enable you to serve your country? I am convinced that a time will come when you will regret not having done what you could. All my hopes are pinned on you and my brother. I had expected that when you grew up, you would enter a trade or profession and serve your unfortunate country at least in a small way. But all in vain! Your only ambition is for the silver shackle. Yes, that is what I call it. What one gets for selling one's freedom for a small sum of money and cutting off all escape is nothing but a legal shackle. A job! I am surprised that you should give in to despair! You have a long life and ample opportunities to decide what work to do. Some among our clever rulers have convinced us that we are not born to be free or to fight the English; and some fools believe it. So long as Indians treat ambition and pride like poison, India will not prosper. There are many among us who despise and abuse the English behind their backs, but bow before them, who despise the opportunity they offer but give fulsome praise for it. But is there any one among us who will extend a helping hand to our country which is drowning? One should learn what is good from the Westerners, and prove one's ability by getting the benefit of their knowledge. Education has become a pretence and an expense with us. It has become a meaningless thing which leads . . . to an empty and false pride. The proper utilisation of the education one has received is . . . an important task entrusted to us by Mother India, and a wanton or deliberate neglect of this duty would make us guilty in the eyes of God. I do not talk about political power, but our people are incapable of doing work which needs courage and thought. What does this show us about the real condition of the people except their slavery? What would society benefit from those who are unenlightened, unable to form an independent opinion, and lack the means of self-defence? And what good influence would be exerted on society by those who are ill-educated, who deserve only to be confined, and who are bound to misuse any concession or kindness offered to them? By what do these people (who are no better than animals) sing the praises of the venerable Aryans? Oh, poor India! You have much to suffer. When will your children wake up and when will their pride be aroused? The world-famous Aryans of yore have now been reduced to the useless Hindus hiding in corners! Will we see even in our dreams the Aryans who conquered all nations of the world and extracted tribute from them? Oh, what a wretched state! Our people grasp the very hand which strikes them and cling to the very foot which kicks them. It is not enough that India is overrun by the English and the missionaries, and has to suffer from their deceit and caprice. There are also hosts of enemies within who are destroying lives and morals. Our truthfulness and uprightness are overshadowed by sin. Our desires, pride, ambition are all suppressed. Our courage and energy have disappeared altogether. We have become suspicious of our real benefactors, we have started to accuse our good advisers of undue interference and political expediency, and we are caught in the net of the enemies whom we heartily embrace. What next? It doesn't need a great astrologer to foretell a terrible disaster. A little thought and consideration will suffice.

You know as well as I do that it was not my duty to apologise to Mr James for whatever my husband did. He knew whether he was doing right or wrong, I bear no responsibility in the matter. And for me to apologise to those who follow their own wishes would be sheer interference. Mr James treated me with kindness, and I will consider him my friend until I hear anything to the contrary. I remember whatever Mr James did for me and am duly thankful to him. But my dear brother-in-law, you ask me to do what I cannot possibly do. You fear that if I don't do it, there will be awkwardness between you and our benefactor Mr James, but this fear is futile and baseless. My idea of friendship might be very different from yours. If friendship is obtained at the cost of independence and freedom of thought, then I firmly believe that the sooner it breaks down the better for both the parties concerned. If friendship is not based on mutual trust, purity of heart and respect, it is better to do without it. If I don't tell you what I think and don't criticise you whenever necessary, I would be failing in my duty to a friend. And if Mr James had not advised my husband the way he did (and that itself was an excellent test of his friendship), I would not have respected him as a friend. But Mr James proved his true and sincere friendship. Now, whether Mr Joshee behaved accordingly is another question.

Should you remain steadfast in your thinking and future plans, and really wish to be a petty clerk or master in the Post Office, do let me know, so that I can write to Mr James about giving you some such position. But I still think that you should make yourself more useful. Tomorrow I will return to Philadelphia. Write to me at that address.[2]

*

It was during this Christmas break that Anandibai wrote her thesis on 'Obstetrics among the Aryan Hindoos' and submitted it to the WMCP for the degree of Doctor of Medicine. Cultural nationalism, which had underpinned all Anandibai's beliefs, also prompted the topic for her dissertation. Having had sporadic contact with missionary schools, she had also been exposed to the racial-cultural superiority of the West and constant criticism of things Indian. Years earlier she had conveyed to Mrs Carpenter (15 November 1880) her determination to study Sanskrit to show the contemptuous Europeans 'how sublime, useful and instructive are the precepts in Hindu shastras'. Her thesis was but an elaboration of some of these 'useful and instructive' precepts. It came at a time when the European 'discovery' of traditional Indian medicine was being lauded. The *Mahratta* (25 October 1885) had boasted:

> European writers have not been slow to recognise the comparative advancement of ancient Hindu medicine, and it is interesting to read in a review of the Standard of the new edition of the British Pharmacopoeia such a passage as this: 'It is certainly true that in the Materia Medica the grandeur of the early empirical knowledge still overshadows the more recent achievements of scientific research. The metals, for instance, which were much more familiarly known in the ancient Hindu medicine than they have been since, are second to no class of remedies in the whole "Pharmacopoeia".'

The extent of Anandibai's own belief in the Ayurvedic school of medicine is unclear, but it should be borne in mind that during her last illness, she was under Ayurvedic treatment, allegedly at her own insistence.

Given the Indian preoccupation with women's reproductive rather than general health, Anandibai's choice of topic was obvious, and may have been reinforced by her own constant ill health and the loss of her infant. It is worth noting that even four decades later, when British medical opinion listed the 'chief objects of women's medical work in India', the priority was given to the safety of Indian women in childbirth, the rest being ranked in the following order: the recognition and treatment of antenatal disease; the training of nurses and midwives; and infant welfare, household hygiene, and research work.[3]

Earlier, in a letter to Mrs Carpenter (6 August 1881) Anandibai had given a brief and cheerful account of Maharashtrian customs surrounding childbirth and the joyous naming ceremony. A contemporary of Anandibai, Yashodabai Joshi, has also left an account of the pampering the new mother receives.

However, there was a grim side to this reality, which *Kesari* had only hinted at: dark, unventilated lying-in rooms, the use of powdered pepper, and filthy midwives. A far more graphic and detailed description was to be provided later by Katherine Mayo in her *Mother India* (1929), where she spoke of substances like powdered pepper inserted into the vagina to expedite delivery; and poor and unskilled low-caste midwives (the only ones who would undertake the 'polluting' job), who would use their unwashed hands with dirt-encrusted nails for the job and who would sometimes use inexpert force and rough handling, adding to the mother's suffering and endangering the infant's life and well-being. Perhaps enough had already been said in and outside India about these practices to put Anandibai on the defensive, for it is precisely these impressions that she seeks to correct.

That Anandibai's thesis was a nationalistic project of retrieving ancient Hindu knowledge was obvious from the very title. The emphasis on 'Aryan' Hindus was a clear statement of cultural nationalism. The term 'Aryan', with its suggestion of a superior race akin to the Europeans, was much in vogue – as seen from Swami Dayanand's 'Arya Samaj', which sought to revive a purified form of Hinduism; Keshub Chunder Sen's Arya Nari Samaj in Bengal, and perhaps based on the same model, Pandita Ramabai's 'Arya Mahila Samaj'. Anandibai herself had indulged in sufficiently stirring rhetoric (in her letter to her brother-in-law written at exactly the same time as her thesis) on the ancient world-renowned Aryans and their present degenerate descendants. In her thesis, her two-pronged attempt was to reinstate ancient Indian medical lore as of equal or greater worth than contemporary Western medicine, and to reconstruct a family and community structure which was far superior to the one then in existence in India (and viewed as corrupted).

*

The opening passage of the thesis very cleverly establishes the long history and tradition of Indian medical science, indirectly suggesting the relative newness of Western medical thought and practice:

As the importance of obstetrics can be measured only by the value of life and health, and both being of paramount consequence, it is deserving of most careful study. When we realise how difficult and vast the subject is, it is not surprising to find so many great minds thoroughly absorbed in its magnitude, from time immemorial. Since our study naturally embraces the cause and effect, race habits, climatic influences and means of assisting Nature in her operations, we must not entirely overlook the history of past ages and consider the superior minds which laboured, with marked success in the same field of investigation, under the promptings of the same motives, as far back as [the] 15th century B.C. they may enable us to the better appreciation of the science and pay due respect to the discoveries, theories and mode of application of remedies of minds of different nations at different times. I therefore need not apologise for choosing this subject.

Beginning with the signs of pregnancy, Anandibai establishes the high level of skill possessed by traditional doctors – the kinds of skills which were ridiculed by Western doctors – and established their legitimacy by citing personal experience: 'I have known at least two native physicians positively decide pregnancy from the pulse alone while in one case of personal acquaintance, there was no other sign present'.

The thesis then goes on to describe the 'hygiene of pregnancy' and the 'good rules . . . laid down by Manu, the great Aryan legislator, Susruta, and other physiologists' whose transgression meant 'committing a sin'. The emphasis throughout is on the meticulous rules of hygiene so valued in the West, and also on the physical and emotional nurturance of the mother-to-be, probably in order to counteract the terrible reports of the actual treatment and misery of Indian women in such a situation in many cases. The gist of the hygiene of pregnancy described by Anandibai is a list of the many ways in which the expecting woman is to be kept safe, secure, and cheerful in terms of her physical, mental, and emotional milieu. She also takes great care to suggest that the current Western interest in eugenics had been anticipated in India centuries earlier.

In order to reinstate the traditional Indian physician, an 'ideal type' description follows: he should be 'of a good family, of a healthy body, young (or old experienced one when a family physician), handsome, pure, vigorous, modest, discreet, patient, firm and intelligent', as well as adept in his profession, dignified, well-mannered, 'gentle, kind, amiable, cheerful' and self-confident. This is matched by a description of the ideal patient: one who follows the physician's instructions, and places her confidence in the physician.

Among the common causes of miscarriage in the nineteenth century, venereal diseases ranked high, as they presumably did in ancient times. Anandibai lists the traditional cures for these as being still effective.

The most important section was the actual confinement – a controversial issue in connection with India. Here a contradiction is apparent between the traditionally recommended and actually used dark room, and the modern preference (shared by Anandibai) for a sunny and airy room. The necessary equipment – hot water, clean clothes for the mother and child, the necessary oils and medicines – should be available from the seventh month onward. The emphasis is on natural delivery, with minimum intervention to be restricted to emergencies.

On the whole, the picture presented is that of the involvement of the family, the nurturance of the expecting mother, especially during her first pregnancy, and meticulous hygienic precautions. At the same time, considerations of 'modesty' proper in women are specified, such as the exclusion of men (other than the physician when necessary) and children as well as young women from the whole process. The dissertation then describes the 'accidents of labour', such as a breach presentation, which might necessitate the performance of a surgical procedure, such as cranioctomy.

Anandibai frequently cites the personal experience of acquaintances to corroborate ancient practices to stress their applicability over time. Thus this American-trained doctor vouches for traditional Indian medicine both from this position of superiority as well as from an insider's experience.

The care of the new mother and the physical examination, care, and diet of the newborn then follows. If a wet nurse needs to be employed, her characteristics are described. Finally, there is a discussion of the diseases common in infancy and their Ayurvedic cures.

She concludes that she is prevented by the scarcity of time and space from doing justice to 'what is taught and practised among the Brahmins'. The thesis was a balancing act: Anandibai carefully selects only the 'many valuable things' – those details which compared well with current Western medical knowledge, and some of which she could personally corroborate, while leaving out the 'many ridiculous ones'.

*

Anandibai's effort to retrieve ancient Indian medical knowledge was among the very first on record. The pioneer in the field was the prolific Dr Sakharam Arjun Raut, Professor of Botany at the Grant Medical College of Mumbai and the stepfather of Dr Rakhmabai, who became Western India's first woman doctor after the early death of Anandibai. He wrote on a variety of medical subjects, aiming to popularise medical knowledge. Most of his books were written in Marathi, and included *The Principles of Medical Science* (1869), which combined Western medicine with ancient Sanskrit texts; *Obstetrics* (1873), which relied on Western books only; *Knowledge of Married Life* (1877); and *The disease of Small-pox, Its Cure and Prevention* (1876).[4] He also wrote *A Catalogue of the Bombay Drugs* in English, giving 'a complete list of the native drugs to be found in the Bazars of Bombay', with their botanical and vernacular names.[5] It would appear, however, that Anandibai was not familiar with any of these publications.

In addition to reclaiming ancient Hindu knowledge, Anandibai also placed it before an international medical forum. That Anandibai's interest in Ayurvedic medicine transcended mere nationalistic pride into genuine faith in its efficacy is suggested by the fact that she was later to undergo Ayurvedic treatment. Had she lived longer, she might even have been able to gradually enter this field, which was guarded by orthodox men. She was the pioneering woman doctor of India, and could have been the pioneering doctor who combined modern Western and traditional Indian medical systems and thus anticipated by a hundred years the current efforts in that direction.

*

After returning from Roselle to Philadelphia, Anandibai was at once caught up in her preparations for the final examination to be held March 1886, followed by an internship. The earlier plan to spend the summer with the Carpenters had to be cancelled because of a special offer of a six-month internship form the New England Hospital for Women and Children at Boston. On 31 January 1886 she wrote to Mrs Carpenter:

My dear Aunt,
    Your disappointment in my change of plans is not greater than mine. I had planned for four months ahead from March. I had forty and one things to finish or accomplish before my hospital service began. But things rotated, no doubt, for our best. I found I must enter the New England hospital next May. You know I have given up Blockley entirely, but will try the competitive for the Woman's Hospital for six months. The friends and authorities of the New England Hospital are very kind to me. They have made special arrangements for me to go there for six months, which is not generally allowable at all. Besides, my application went too late, all the places were filled, yet they are so anxious to help me, that they are going to accept me as an extra student or interne. Such students pay board, but they make me their guest. Dr Tyng is also willing to take me for six months provided I pass the competitive. Now everything depends on my graduating. If faithful attendance and diligent study with some practical knowledge deserve any

reward at all, I have no reason to fear next March, but I have to wait for it.

Do not buy me anything for my graduation. Your presence will make me more happy than any gift. It is not as if I had no memento; but nothing can be added. If you were troubled with wealth, I would accept anything you might present me. Now I hope you will present yourselves, which is the richest of gifts.

I had the misfortune to fall on the ice and break all the bangles on my right arm [hand]. My husband bought me a gold bracelet, as I could not go without anything. If every fall would bring as much gold, would you consider it a misfortune? I called it so, because the money might have bought me an instrument that would have been useful or a book that would have been instructive. I got another present as a graduating student, five weeks in advance. It is a beautiful gold watch. It was given me by a wealthy lady, whom you will probably see in March.

Our theses, ticket money, and application for degree were sent in last week. I do not yet know whether my 'Thesis' is accepted. There were fifty pages of it, just fitting, so that not another word could have gone in; the longest one they had.[6]

By this time Anandibai's health seemed to be delicate, and she seemed to have lost courage. Her performance could no longer match in quality that of the first two years in college. On 8 February she wrote to Mrs Carpenter:

Love and duty are sacred and <u>my own</u>. I can always love, although I cannot always expect to be loved. So I can always perform my own duty, although I may not persuade others to perform theirs. I do not do this for the promise of any earthly pleasure, nor even for those termed heavenly, but for simple duty's sake. Heaven, if it be only a place of indulgence and banqueting, would have no charm for me for these might disappear and leave me paralysed and idle. It is always well to look into the future just far enough to guide our steps and prepare for any immediate obstruction, but I think it is foolish, if not worse, to mourn over the possible future when the present needs all our watchfulness and strength. My physical self is like the days of September, and my brain and nerves seem 'dissected up' like the warp on the loom, distinct and bare, but sensitive.[7]

*

Meanwhile, developments in India, such as the setting up of the Dufferin Fund, caught up with Anandibai, and she received a job offer soon after her final examination. As an extension of the Dufferin scheme, the princely state of Kolhapur in the Bombay Presidency had opened the Edward Albert Memorial Hospital on 3 July 1884 (as an addition to the original hospital, opened in 1851), 'a magnificent building in the Gothic style' named after the Prince of Wales, whose visit to India it intended to commemorate. The state authorities were prepared to open 'a class for female medical pupils', assisting them with stipends and a promise of financial support if they did well enough to enter the Grant Medical College at Mumbai.[8] A woman doctor was also to be invited from abroad to take charge of the proposed female ward.

The Dewan of Kolhapur had already written to Dean Bodley, towards the end of 1885, in search of an American lady doctor for the state, when he heard from Justice Ranade that Anandibai would soon qualify herself. Obviously a Maharashtrian lady doctor would be eminently suitable, and Dean Bodley was requested to convey the offer to Anandibai, along with the terms and conditions which were quite reasonable. She was offered a contract for seven years (to be terminated by either party with a six months' notice) from 1 June 1886, at a joining monthly salary of Rs 300, to be increased to Rs 400 after two years of service, and to Rs 500 after five years. A house with ordinary furniture, but without service or board, would be provided for her use. Her passage from the United States to Kolhapur would be paid, to be refunded if she left the service in less than a year. Anandibai was to be in charge of the Edward Albert Hospital under the general supervision of the State Doctor (one Dr Sinclair), and instruct a class of girls in medicine. These girls were to be trained in Mumbai to be general practitioners; they were to be allotted quarters near Mrs Joshee's. Ladies of the palace and wives of contributors to the Hospital Funds were to be treated free of charge, and private practice would be allowed as long as it did not interfere with hospital duties. Provided Anandibai responded favourably, she was to write a letter to that effect.[9]

Anandibai accepted the appointment cordially, making the point that she considered medical help as a social service and not a lucrative source of income; thus, if she charged a fee at all, it would be from 'those who are rich and powerful, and never from those who are poor and depressed'.[10]

There were other similar requests for a lady doctor from India. Before the Kolhapur offer was finalised, Dr Bodley had considered an offer from Ahmedabad, which offered very similar terms and conditions. The identity of the institution on whose behalf the offer was made is not clear.

*

The news of Anandibai's appointment was duly announced and welcomed at a public meeting in Mumbai on 31 March 1886, as reported by the *Mahratta* (4 April 1886). The efforts of the Regent of Kolhapur who, after a personal interview with the Queen during his visit to England, had resolved to appoint a lady doctor in Kolhapur and start medical classes for women, were described amid cheers. Dr Bodley's reply to a query about Anandibai was also read aloud and well received, especially her revelation that she had passed her examinations 'creditably, ranking eighth in her class which consists of forty-two ladies' and that she had good prospects of completing her examinations in March 1886. As to her character and ability, 'the popular estimate is most favourable': 'She is modest, dignified, and prudent, and she has won the hearts of all those associated with her by her steadfast devotion to duty. She dresses as a Hindu lady, and abstains wholly from animal food'.

Two letters were cited, written to Lady Reay, wife of the Governor of Bombay, who had taken charge of the Bombay scheme for Female Medical Education – one by a friend in Philadelphia and another by Ramabai Ranade, both lauding Anandibai. The meeting was concluded on a laudatory note by the British speaker:

> Surely this spectacle of a young Brahman lady . . . going to the other end of the world to study medicine; living alone among a strange people, but retaining her own national dress, and her own religion and special customs, devoting herself to study, but finding time to cultivate the friendship of those about her, and to win their affection and esteem; supporting herself the while on a scholarship won by her own exertion; surely, I say, such a spectacle justified the creed of those who believe, as I do, that the women of this country are capable of receiving, and ready to receive, the highest education, and that if their fathers and their husbands and their brothers will only give them encouragement, we shall in a few years have an abundant supply of native ladies, holding medical diplomas and practising their profession with profit to themselves and advantage to their countrywomen in every town in the Presidency. Sceptics may say that Mrs Joshi's [sic] case is an exceptional and solitary one, and that one swallow does not make a spring. I reply that it is not so.

Notes

1 Kanitkar, pp. 78–82.
2 Ibid, p. 82, my translation.

3 Scharlieb, Mary "Foreword" to *The Work of Medical Women in India* by Balfour, Margaret I. and Young, Ruth, 1929, New York: OUP, p. xi.
4 Mohini Varde, *Dr. Rakhmabai Ek Aart*, (Marathi Edition) (Marathi) Paperback, Popular Publication 1982, p. 188.
5 Ibid, p. 189.
6 Dall, pp. 125–26.
7 Ibid, p. 127.
8 *Mahratta*, 13 July 1884.
9 Dall, pp. 143–44.
10 Ibid, p. 146.

13

GRADUATION AND AFTER

The grand and glittering occasion when the thirty-three students of the Woman's Medical College of Pennsylvania's class of 1886, visibly dominated by Anandibai, graduated, was to serve multiple agendas for its diverse participants. For Anandibai, herself, the climactic completion of her medical course was a personal triumph and a partial fulfilment of her nationalist and feminist commitment to her compatriot women. For the WMCP authorities it was their widely publicised contribution to the education of women from diverse countries, and in Anandibai's well-publicised case, also to the welfare and eventual emancipation of Indian women across the globe. But the Indo-American connection had other and wider repercussions: The occasion was to serve as the platform from which Pandita Ramabai's career as a feminist ideologue and practitioner was to be launched. It is difficult today to adequately appreciate the uniqueness of having two Indian women in the United States at the same moment at a time when Indian women were highly troped as confined to the domestic sphere and when even Indian men rarely went abroad, especially to America.

Ramabai, who was to claim the lion's share of the limelight trained on Anandibai, had been specially invited by Dr Bodley from England to attend the graduation, or 'commencement'. Bodley later reminisced that the two women, though 'kinswomen', 'never met until they greeted each other under my roof, March 6th, 1886; but, as kindred spirits, they had corresponded for several years'.[1] This was true only in a symbolic sense; their first meeting actually took place at the wharf in Philadelphia where Anandibai had rushed to receive Ramabai in a state of near exhaustion almost as soon as her final examinations were over, as she described to Mrs Carpenter on 7 March 1886:

Dear Aunt,
    At last I am able to sit down at my ease and write to my dear ones. I am through the studies as far as college life is

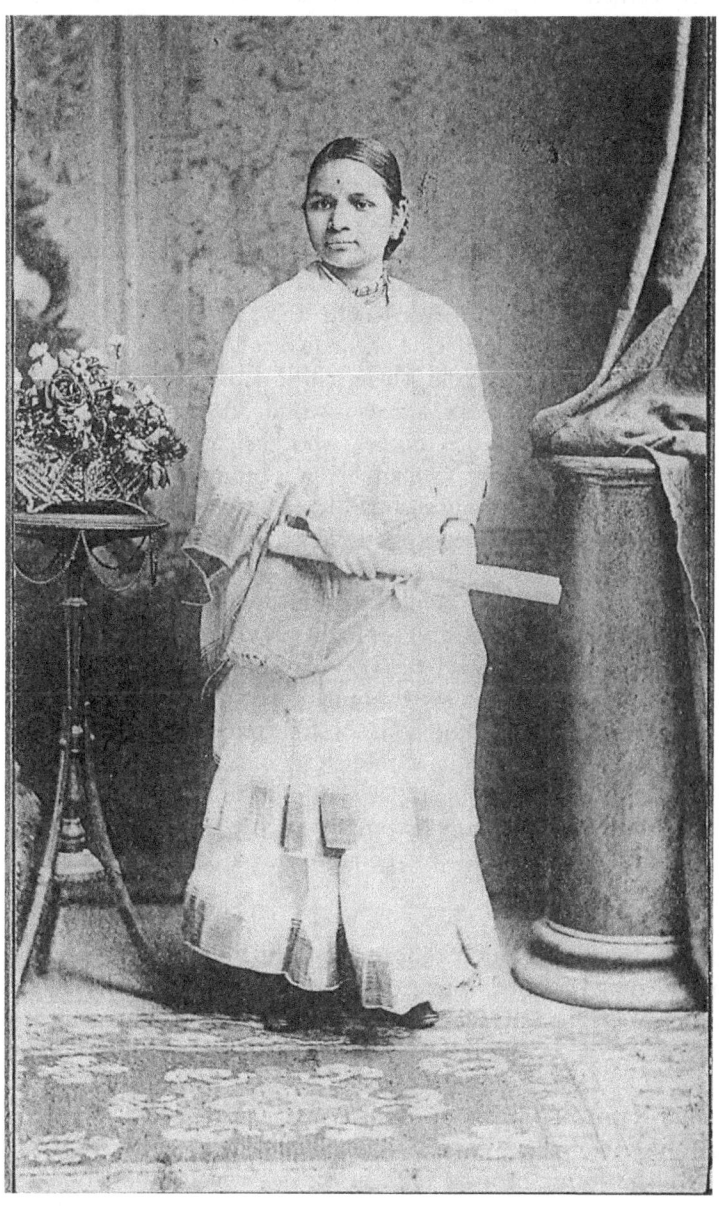

Figure 13.1 Anandibai with her medical degree

Source: Courtesy of S. Vaidya

concerned, but, oh dear! There is so much that comes after than goes before.

Results received yesterday and I have passed. I am thankful, for my patience was almost worn out. On the last question of my last paper I almost broke down, and could not even see whether I finished my sentence. I pinned the papers together and left the room without even bowing to the Professor. Our Japanese friend did very well. The [ungrateful] Syrian student . . . was made to leave us. Her condition is sadder than death, if death is at all sad. . . . .

Pandita Ramabai arrived safely. The storm and low water detained her in the river. I spent two full days on the wharf waiting for her. Her child is here, a little darling. She is as bright as sunshine and sweet as a fresh rosebud. She must give a great deal of comfort to her mother, who has passed through too many sorrows for one woman. She was brought up and petted by sensitive and loving hearts. She is a woman, tender with feelings, as tender as a flower, timid as can be and impatient of pain, but her courage has outweighed that of the sternest and bravest warrior. She has filled my heart with a real joy. I hope you will like her when you see her.

I began to write this letter yesterday, but so much else came in the way! I went to my Examination at the College at 7:45 this morning, and came home at 2:40 p.m. The examination was very long and tedious, though it could not be considered hard. I did not have much sleep last night and I was very tired; am so tired I can hardly keep my eyes open or my hand under control. I am glad you are going to stay a day longer for the lecture of Ramabai.[2]

Mrs Carpenter's greatest concern was for the ill effects the exhausted Anandibai had suffered from exposure to the cold winds on the wharf.[3] But Anandibai herself seemed to be impervious to it in her excitement.

*

Pandita Ramabai's arrival on the scene was no accident, but rather a part of Dean Bodley's carefully framed strategy to garner support for Anandibai's future medical work in India – when job offers were yet to come and when her medical career seemed uncertain. Familiar with Ramabai's reputation as the acknowledged champion of Indian women's education, she had written to Ramabai at Cheltenham on 28 December 1885:

My thought in inviting you to come to America early in 1886 has been that if the tidings might be sent to India that you braved a wintry ocean to witness Anandibai receive her degree as a Doctor of Medicine, you in a certain sense gave your sanction to her act and enfolded her and her work in your future leadership.[4]

Ramabai herself had reached a kind of dead-end in her career trajectory in England and welcomed the opportunity, although the Anglican sisters at Wantage opposed her plan. Possibly, Anandibai had played a direct role in managing the invitation.

To an unimagined extent, Ramabai's visit caused a stir in the United States. The *New York Times* reproduced a full report from the *Philadelphia Ledger* about 'the distinguished Brahmin lady', underscoring the Brahmin mystique. Mrs Dall, having gone to Philadelphia to make her acquaintance, was very favourably impressed. Predictably, her first reaction to Ramabai's light-skinned and grey-eyed beauty was couched in racial terms:

Ramabai is strikingly beautiful. Her face is a clean-cut oval; her eyes, dark and large, glow with feeling. She is a brunette but her cheeks are full of colour. Her white widow's sari is drawn closely over her head and fastened under her chin. There is nothing else about her to suggest the Hindu [i.e. Indian].[5]

Dall was obviously much struck by Ramabai's 'un-Indian' appearance: 'I cross-questioned Anandabai pretty closely about a possible mixture of blood. She acknowledged that there is a frequent crossing of the Mahratta blood by that of Cashmere'.[6] Although this explanation of the fair skin common among Chitpavans sounds highly improbable and was possibly misunderstood by Dall, the foregrounding of the racial angle is significant.

The extent to which Ramabai's appearance contributed to her cordial reception (based primarily on her charismatic personality and Christian orientation) remains a matter of speculation. But a mention of her 'dark' eyes is obviously a racial stereotype: Her eyes were greenish-grey, as described by eyewitnesses and shown by photos.

*

The commencement ceremony on 11 March 1886 was a grand and well-attended affair which filled the city newspapers. Anandibai and Ramabai (described variously as her relative, cousin, and aunt) seemed inadvertently to vie for public attention. The greatest enthusiasm was displayed by the *Philadelphia Evening Bulletin* (11 March 1886), which had prepared the ground in its report with a long rubric: 'Commencement Day: The Woman's Medical College; Thirty-three Women Given the Right to Practice Medicine – Who the Graduates Are – A Distinguished Lady' and given extensive coverage to 'Pandita Ramabai, a distinguished Brahmin lady [who], with her daughter, was present to witness the graduation of her relative, Mrs Anandibai Joshee'. The report detailed Ramabai's efforts in founding the Arya Mahila Samaj and promoting women's education in India, as well as her career in England, emphasising her 'professorship of Sanskrit' (erroneously attributed to Professor Max Mueller's recommendation). The paper also gave (12 March 1886) the most complete account of the ceremony, including the following:

> The feature of yesterday's commencement was the graduation of the native East Indian lady Mrs Anandibai Joshee, who has pursued the full course of study at the Woman's Medical College, and graduates with high honours to go back to the work of ministry among her own sex at home. Mrs Joshee's appearance on the stage yesterday, as she modestly advanced to receive her diploma, was hailed with repeated rounds of hearty applause from the crowded audience, who seemed desirous to add all possible honours to the brave little woman who has thus far accomplished her remarkable undertaking, while her relative, the Pundita Ramabai, who has crossed the ocean from England to witness the event, was present to witness the spirited scene.

In its report, the *Philadelphia Record* (12 March 1886) mentioned an 'important personage' on the stage, the white-clad 'Pundita Ramabai, the distinguished Brahmin lady from Poona, India', who had made the long journey from England for her relative. The *Philadelphia Press* of the same day added:

> Each graduating student was greeted with applause as she stepped on the stage, and little Mrs Joshee, the Indian lady, who graduated with high honours in her class, received quite an ovation. Her native costume, a graceful robe of white linen bordered with gold, was in pronounced contrast against the background of sombre-robed ladies and black-garmented men on the stage. Her husband looked on from a box, and also her

aunt, the widowed Pundita Ramabai, who but recently arrived with her little daughter from England.

Mrs Dall gives a vivid account of the ceremony and the two Indian women who riveted everybody's attention:

> How different they were! One so strikingly beautiful that she arrested every eye, the other self-absorbed, unconscious, with her gaze fixed upon the Highest. One impulsive, practical, bent on carrying out certain plans for the benefit of her people; the other devout, self-controlled, thinking first of all of the great mysteries of life and work . . . although not in the least beautiful, [Mrs Joshee] is the sweetest impersonation of pure womanliness that I have ever seen. All eyes were on her. Ramabai . . . has a really handsome face, a delicate skin flushed with brilliant color. She and her little girl look like Spaniards. Neither is graceful, while every motion of Anandabai gives pleasure . . . Anandabai had many valuable presents, books, instrument/s and money, to help her carry out her purpose. She could hardly be insensible to the fact that she was the observed of all observers; she must have heard the frequent and honourable mention of her name, nor could she have been deaf to the applause of that immense audience when she went forward to take her diploma, but not even the quiver of her lips betrayed her.[7]

The WMCP authorities had been prompt in conveying the news of Anandibai's graduation to Britain, perhaps with a hint at America's having successfully pre-empted Britain in a progressive initiative for Indian women. In reply, Sir Henry Ponsonby, Queen Victoria's Private Secretary, wrote from Windsor on 14 July 1886 to the British legation of the United States:

> I am commanded by the Queen to request that you will kindly thank Dr Bodley for having sent to Her Majesty the account of Dr Joshee's graduation at the Woman's Medical College of Pennsylvania, and to assure you that the Queen has read it with much interest.[8]

*

Pandita Ramabai's address the day after the graduation was reported in detail by the *Philadelphia Evening Bulletin* (13 March 1886) under the rubric 'Pundita Ramabai in America: A Hindoo Widow Talks to

American Women – A unique and striking Scene'. The paper spoke of her as 'a Hindoo woman of high caste, her slight figure wrapped in the white robes of Hindu widowhood, out of which looked a face of most picturesque beauty and expression' addressing 'a large audience and surrounded by fifty or sixty of the best women of Philadelphia'. She delivered her talk in a musical voice, with genuine simplicity and noble sentiments, describing the conditions and needs of Indian women; and ended on an all-inclusive note:

> And when the earnest little lady suddenly closed her address by asking an American company of educated and refined men and women to join with her in a moment's silent prayer 'to the Great Father of all the nations of the earth' in [sic] behalf of the millions of her Hindoo sisters to whose cause she has given her life, there was something almost startling in the strangeness of the unique situation.

Mrs Dall corroborated that an audience of almost six hundred was 'reverent, struck by the speaker's beauty and awed by her enthusiasm and eloquence'. Her final, earnest appeal was followed by a hush and '[t]he whole city echoed the next day with wondering inquiry and explanation'.[9]

That Ramabai and Anandibai operated within entirely different paradigms was obvious from the outset. Anandibai was imbued with the pride of the Hindu culture and her Brahmin lineage, unable or unwilling to admit the problems of Indian women to foreigners. Ramabai had freely 'named' the problem – the multiple oppression of Indian women – in both India and abroad, in the belief that unless you name and analyse the problem, you cannot begin to solve it. Again, as a Christian, Ramabai was at once embraced by American women wholeheartedly.

But on this occasion the differences were elided, because taken together the two Indian women offered an opportunity to strengthen the existing but tenuous relationship between America and India. Medical work often went hand in hand with missionary work, and there was a strong desire to open up the field – generally claimed by Britain as the colonial power – to allow the entry of American women. While introducing Ramabai, Dr Bodley alluded to 'the bridge of womanly sympathy which, beginning with Harriet Newell, seventy-one years ago, had gradually been built across the great chasm between America and India' – the bridge across which there had been travel from West to East, but now the solitary figure of Anandibai had crossed from East to West and was now 'crowned with the fruits of her patient, persistent labour and study, the first native Indian woman' to bear the medical diploma in her country.

*

While critiquing this lionisation of Ramabai, the *Mahratta* (13 March 1886) reproduced Dr Bodley's speech and the part related to Anandibai's long struggle to get her medical degree. The news was predictably greeted with great excitement and admiration in Maharashtra and even *Kesari*, which had opposed the introduction of Western medical health care for women, wholeheartedly supported Anandibai's medical training and future career in India. On 27 April 1886, it published a news item on the Lady Dufferin Fund and its perceived evil effects in aiding and abetting the entry of Christianity into Hindu families, written with heavy sarcasm, which the paper generally reserved for progressive initiatives. Juxtaposed with this was an item extolling Anandibai's efforts and the value of her knowledge for the welfare of Indian women. It suggested that eminent people should start a class for the women of their families for which Anandibai would impart basic medical knowledge against an appropriate salary; and that another course should be started in Marathi to prepare girls for a career as medical doctors or midwives. Importantly,

> Anandibai should not be allowed to take up service in a Native State or with Government. This will not yield the maximum benefit. In our opinion, if an attempt is made to disseminate medical knowledge among our women in this manner, it will become more successful and popular than the efforts made by Lady Dufferin with the help of the entire official machinery.

Monopolising Anandibai's medical expertise for a people's initiative in competition with the colonial state or princely states was *Kesari*'s own brand of nationalism.

*

The much publicised graduation, the culmination of three years of intense effort, was followed by an exhilarating round of social visits and sightseeing excursions for Anandibai, accompanied by Ramabai. It ended with Manorama's illness, through which Anandibai nursed her day and night, falling ill herself. The three of them then went to Roselle for a rest, where Gopalrao and Govindrao Sathe joined them.

Anandibai went to Roxbury, Massachusetts, for her internship. At the New England Hospital she was promised 'ample opportunity to visit other infirmaries and asylums not unfriendly to women' and, instead of 'the care and responsibility devolving upon an interne', 'would give her the chance to see a great variety of work'.[10] Her letter from Roxbury to Mrs Carpenter on 3 May 1886 reported her progress as much as her renewed illness:

> My dear Aunt,
> I reached here last evening at about 7 o'clock. Two of my college friends came very kindly to meet me, so that made it pleasant all through. I have already taken charge of the medical ward here. I went to the Maternity ward to see a case soon after I arrived, before supper. This morning at seven I visited the medical ward. At 8:30 I went with another Interne to the Surgical. I paid another visit at 12:30 with Dr P. this is one of the regular visits.
> I have to visit my own ward again this evening, so you see how busy I am! I have to make three regular visits beside that with Dr P to all the Hospital, after which the consulting physician, resident physician and the Interns meet in the office to discuss the cases. My sleeping-room is on the third floor, dining-room on the lowest, patients all over. I have to fill up the papers that belong to my own patients. This is the first time I have sat down. I am so tired!
> The spot in which the Hospital stands is one of the most delightful that I have seen. It is perfectly charming. It was so cold in the house that I came out on the lawn to write. It is very sunny, but very windy, so I don't think I shall stay long . . .
> Will you please give the Roorhacks my address, and tell them not to send me the knife for wood carving or anything else. I have to be moving from room to room and place to place, and have no time for anything. After all, I have regular duty to perform. One of my college friends has left the Hospital entirely, the other is miles off in the Dispensary.
> You will be sorry to hear that I have such a cold in my throat that I cannot talk, only whisper. There is measles in the Annex, so one interne must stay here. Two others have left. Dr Hall is here, but Dr Sterling has not yet come.
> With love . . .[11]

Soon Anandibai was confined to her room, and on 5 June Mrs Dall was shocked to find her 'lying in bed, pale and quiet'.[12] Hospital work had to be given up, and she planned to return to Roselle by short stages.

On 9 June she mustered enough strength to visit Mrs Underwood, a friend of Mrs Dall's, in Boston for an evening, and meet a few friends. Mrs Underwood's account of the occasion (with the inevitable preoccupation with Anandibai's appearance) sheds an interesting light on Anandibai's sensitivity to foreign critiques of India which stemmed from ignorance and prejudice:

> She wore no bonnet, but instead a fawn-coloured wrap enveloped her finely shaped head and gracefully draped shoulders; this was removed on entering. Her robe of some fine dark woollen material was edged to the depth of several inches with gold-coloured embroidery, and in spite of its flowing drapery at one arm, fitted nicely her plump petite form; gold bracelets adorned her wrists. The dark face was round with full lips; she had a handsomely shaped brow, broad and intellectual looking. Between the eyebrows was a small tattooed mark, in shape somewhat like a cross. The eyes were beautiful and expressive, large, black, softly shining, as capable of smiles as of tears, with a strangely pathetic look in them. The prevailing expression of Dr Joshee's was grave, dignified almost sad, but the rare smile which marked her appreciation of the ludicrous was charmingly bright and girlish. The talk drifted during the evening into channels which in spite of modest diffidence drew her out. The Car of Juggernaut was discussed, and in speaking of the mothers who, distraught with poverty, sometimes throw their babes into the Ganges, Dr Joshee said that during her medical experience in Philadelphia a large number of infants, either murdered or deserted, found their way into the dissecting-room, and she might as well on her return to India relate this fact, making it a custom of American mothers to kill or desert their children, and adducing it as a result of Christian belief, as to charge the Hindu faith with the drowning so often reported.

In discussing the right of men to kill and eat animals, Dr Joshee said that she had lived in America for three years without feeling the need of any other food than that which she ate in India. In speaking of Edwin Arnold's poems, by which she meant the 'Song Celestial' and 'Indian Idylls', she said she had not exaggerated, but sometimes failed to catch, the subtle spiritual meanings of the ancient writings.

She spoke sensibly of 'Christian Science', said she had taken several lessons in that art of healing, and thought she saw a natural basis on which it could be explained. She spoke of phrenology, and said that in dissecting the brain she had found reason to dispute the claims made by its enthusiastic advocates.

Her acquaintance with American and English scientists and persons of note was something phenomenal. As she glanced over a large collection of portrait photographs, a word or two would show that she was familiar with the story of each man and his work.[13]

*

When Anandibai went to Roselle on 1 July 1886, her friends became anxious about her health; but a thorough medical examination does not seem to have been done. On 10 July she left for Delaware County, New York, for a vacation with Eighmie.[14] In mid-July she wrote to Mrs Carpenter that she was enjoying herself:

> We are having lovely times. I have not botonised, but we roam about and work. Sometimes we find nice little strawberry patches and we eat of the fruit heartily. The day before yesterday Eighmie and I went to Aunt Jenny's. I took my 'crazy' work with me, and made one block.[15]

The 'crazy work' was a patchwork quilt with different blocks or squares contributed by her American friends, and finally to be finished at Roselle.[16] Already on 20 July Anandibai wrote again to Mrs Carpenter to say that she was cutting short her vacation because of ill health.

> How I wish you were here. I won't stay much longer, for I have been ill ever since I came. I am having chills three times a day, and fever. My whole body is aching. If you do not come within a reasonable time, I shall leave this place and go to you. I am afraid I shall not see you much before I go to India.[17]

On 23 July followed another letter from Anandibai, with more distressing news regarding her health: 'I am now having two chills daily, and fever after each one. My throat is so inflamed that it keeps me coughing all the time. Last night I did not have five minutes' rest'.[18]

*

Meanwhile, India continued to beckon. On 13 July 1886 came a letter from the Dewan of Kolhapur (dated 12 June 1886), enclosing a resolution from the proceedings of the Council of Administration held on 7 June 1886, confirming Anandibai's appointment and requesting details of her plans to sail for India.

200

Having been compelled by ill health to give up her internship at Roxbury, Anandibai turned her attention to her duties in India. These included family matters in addition to her new post; and she wrote first to her mother-in-law and then a brother-in-law suggesting that they join her at Kolhapur as soon as she reached it. She also mentioned in the latter letter that she might travel alone to India via England, because Gopalrao was uncertain about joining her, making excuses for staying on for a few months. He seemed to have developed an interest in Russia and also wished to visit England and 'abuse the people there'. In the same letter she mentions having been treated successfully by a couple of doctors for her chills and fever, and finally having started taking 'her own' medicine, which had promising results.[19]

Anandibai seemed to accept without a murmur Gopalrao's abdication of his family obligations, and assumed the financial and practical responsibility of providing for her marital family in a reversal of roles. Her letter to her brother-in-law offers the very first, and rare, hint of her impatience with his disregard for her welfare and his self-centred travel plans, and especially with his obsession with publicly criticising the English society. His similar behaviour in America had already caused her untold embarrassment.

*

Gopalrao had made considerable waves on the American scene, having lost no opportunity to engage in debates and to uphold Hindu culture as superior to American. In a letter sent from Philadelphia in mid-March and published in the *Index* (1 April 1886) of Boston, he championed the Indian custom of child marriage:

In your issue of the 11*th* inst., child marriages are put forth as abominations. Why? Because they are simple and innocent. Child marriages are abominations because of our abhorrence for the lottery in love. If people would be satisfied with late or choice marriages, I would not condemn them. But there is a system whereby marriages are made and unmade according to the demands of lust. India abounds in civilised people who adopt this substitute for early and permanent marriage. We do not want that cheap commodity from Europe. Let England and America preserve it as an emblem of independence and liberty. . . . In every part of India, not to speak of the Native States, child marriages are performed and celebrated by hundreds and thousands every year, under the very noses of the men who rule over us. . . . Wherever child marriage does not prevail, there prostitution is carried on, on an extensive scale. . . . [The spouses married in childhood] when they come of age, live so peacefully and harmoniously that they are never separated. We have no such divorce system as you have in the United States. . . .

In conclusion, I beg you, dear Editors, never to say a word against my country. We have no confidence in your careless press, unprincipled missionaries, crafty politicians, and cunning presidents. The Americans have no shining character to boast of to other nations. . . . We don't want your marriage system. We don't want your divorce. We don't want your swindles and frauds. Keep them all to yourselves. We don't envy you. But don't condemn our child marriage system and call us by hard names.

The letter not only was placed at the head of the correspondence column, but also drew a somewhat defensive response, published below it, which dealt with five of the points raised by Gopalrao. This was to herald a close association between him and the newspaper. A few months later the *Index* (10 June 1886) reported on a debate on religion at which Gopalrao was introduced as 'not . . . a member of the Brahmo Samaj, or of Reformed Hinduism, but . . . an adherent of the ancient Brahmanism'. His address on 'What is Lacking in Christianity' was liberally sprinkled with 'substantiated' statements that Christianity lacked justice, righteousness, humanity, honesty of purpose, and charity. It concluded:

Though Christianity does not possess any noble attribute, yet this country is most prosperous and wealthy. As I said before, Christianity is the best fertilizer, but a most disgusting thing to look at.

The address had a remarkably indulgent reception from the president at the debate who advocated introspection for Christians in the same issue of the paper:

If there are any Christians of the Evangelical type in this hall, perhaps they now begin to understand how a pagan may feel when he hears his religion characterized by an Orthodox Christian. Mr Joshee has turned the tables. This is the way Christendom looks to his unsophisticated eyes. It will do us no harm to reflect on the picture, and there are lessons which we may well take to heart in his drawing of it, though it does not flatter Christian pride.

Gopalrao's latest outburst when Anandibai wrote to her brother-in-law had been in June, in an address he gave at Concord, Massachusetts, on 'Missionaries in India', subsequently published in the *Index* (22 July 1886). After 'giving praise where praise is due' and acknowledging that the 'disinterested philanthropy' of the missionaries 'has awakened all nations to their sense of duty and responsibility', he launched into an attack:

> These greedy Christians did not go into the adjoining countries where there was nothing but sand and flint, but to those countries which abounded in gold and silver, and where industry was an honest pursuit and selfishness an unpardonable sin, and ingratitude a capital crime. . . . the so-called missionaries are sappers and miners. They go first to cut trees and make roads, and close behind them are the army and warships. In the recent China-French trouble, the missionaries are found to be the political spies.
>
> Now ninety-nine per cent of the people who contribute to support the so-called missionaries are entirely in the dark as to what they have been doing in foreign lands. If they were to know one-hundredth part of the mischief done by the missionaries, they would stand aghast for the part they have unknowingly taken in the massacre of mankind and the general immoral education imparted to them. . . .
>
> In Burmah and Japan no locks and keys are in use. Doors are open day and night, but in Christian countries door have as many bolts and locks as there are members in the house. Christians manufactured all the vices, and exported those commodities to foreign lands where simplicity and innocence reigned. So, your drunkenness is the Christian blessing or salvation conferred on the children of India. England and America are the boasted nations of the universe, and yet they are the most unscrupulous and unprincipled. I do not speak against Christ and his teachings, but I find his followers unworthy of the name. I have been with missionaries for the last twenty-two years. The more I look into their characters, the darker is the dye that stains them. . . . Christians have manufactured all the vices, and exported them to countries where simplicity and innocence reigned.[20]

In substantiation of his charges, Gopalrao revealed the missionary strategy during Anandibai's voyage to America, to force her to eat meat so that she would lose caste and be prepared to accept Christianity. Mrs Dall, unaware of the incident, was particularly incensed by this address because of help she knew had been given to Anandibai by missionaries, and asked Gopalrao if he thought that her missionary husband, Mr Dall, also fitted the description. Gopalrao disclaimed any knowledge of Mr Dall; but a month later, when the news of Mr Dall's death in India was received, he condoled with her, saying that she could not imagine 'how much he was beloved in India'. Anandibai sat by him 'throughout his long tirade, silent and suffering'.[21]

About August 1886, Anandibai wrote again to her mother-in-law from Roselle, and aired her homesickness:

> I am longing to have a good meal in India. This country has hardly anything worth eating. These people do not know how to cook. Rice is boiled in knee-deep water and still remains only half-cooked. All in all, it is a . . .?? of all dishes. Anyway one has to make do with what one gets. I will not recover unless I get a good square meal with lentil curry, vegetables and *bhakri*. You will laugh at my crazy babbling. Pray send your reply to Roselle by return of post; otherwise I will have left. I am enclosing some flowers; please keep them if you like, or else give them to Bapu [Ketkar?] if he wants them.[22]

*

Earlier in August, Anandibai went to Rochester, New York, to meet Gopalrao, who had preceded her, and wrote to Mrs Carpenter on 10 August:

> I arrived at the station at 9:05 p.m. and at this place at 10:10 p.m. I had a very pleasant and comfortable journey. I was not at all sick, and did not cough more than six or seven times. I was not at all hungry, and ate nothing until 7 o'clock. Mr Joshee did not come to meet me in time, but it was not his fault. I wrote him that the train arrived at 9:55, so he did not start till after I had arrived. I inquired at the station and took the tramway near it. I told the conductor where I wanted to go. He told me where to change cars and where to walk on the street. Every house was dark and I could not tell where I was.
>
> Finally I found some people sitting on a piazza and asked them what number their house bore. They said seventy, so I turned and went back. Mr Joshee came in forty minutes after

I found the house. I had a terrible coughing spell in the street car. I found a white piece which I thought was five cents, and dropped it in. the good driver looked in the box and asked me if I had put in some money. I said, Yes, when he showed me that I had put in 25 cents. He was very sorry, and so was I, but I did not say anything. The honest driver could not open the box, but he managed so nicely that I got twenty cents back. A gentleman who stepped in was told by the driver of my mistake and paid me his fare; nor did the driver let anybody put in another fare till I had my twenty cents back. I could not help feeling extremely grateful to the stranger for his kindness. My impression is that the drivers are honest. This is the way I have always found people.

I can't write any better and cough too.[23]

On the health front, things went steadily from bad to worse, although Anandibai continued to make detailed travel plans to visit as many parts of the United States as possible, often at the invitation of her friends. Her next letter to Mrs Carpenter from Rochester on 18 August 1886 was dictated to a companion:

My dear Aunt,

Your letters are at hand. Dr Bodley is not able to go with me, so I shall leave for the Falls on the 20*th*. Mr Joshee will go with me as far as the Falls. He will put [me] in the car/s for Chicago, where my friend will meet me. She will show me everything worth seeing in that city. From Chicago I will buy a ticket to Warrensburg, Missouri, where Dr Smith will meet me. I shall leave Dr Smith to go to Cincinnati, where I shall meet Dr Bodley. Will you be kind enough to send my red silk saree which is in the trunk, and either my shawl or my graduating dress? My friends are so disappointed that I have not any pretty dresses with me! And Dr Smith wants me to bring some pretty sarees. They will not get lost if they are expressed. My cough is not any better. Love to all.[24]

However, Dr Bodley changed her plans to suit Anandibai's convenience and joined her, together with Ramabai, at Rochester. The proposed journey had to be cut short, and new plans were made to visit only Niagara Falls. From there the company decided to return to Philadelphia, because, as Anandibai wrote to Mrs Dall, she did not have much strength left – although there was no need to worry.[25] On the way to

Philadelphia the party broke journey at Carlisle, at Anandibai's express wish to visit the school for American Indian youth. Then she continued to Philadelphia and spent ten days at the Woman's Hospital to rest and receive treatment.[26] Her health was precarious, as she wrote to Mrs Dall:

> Even the least breeze seems to abuse me. No one in the house realises the trouble as my Doctor and I do, and no one need. My headache, which is reflex, is perfectly intolerable. It is aggravated by every attempt to think.[27]

From Philadelphia Anandibai went with Ramabai to Roselle, where she spent her last month in America, debilitated but in good spirits, as described by Mrs Carpenter:

> Her strength was so far reduced that during the four weeks that she remained with us, the greater part of the time was spent in bed or on the lounge though she generally joined us at lunch or dinner. With her husband, her cousin, and Mr Sattay [sic] in the house, there was everything to make her last days here as comfortable as her condition would allow, and in the merry social converse, in which she eagerly joined, she would have forgotten that she was an invalid, had it not been for the frequent and periodical taking of medicine.
>
> At no time did any of the 'gloom' of the sick room attend her. Everything was done to make those precious days as bright and cheerful as possible. It was too hard to believe that all the efforts of her physicians would be in vain, and we tried to shut our eyes to the heart-rending truth.[28]

It was under these conditions that preparations were made for Anandibai and Gopalrao's journey to India, and her eleven trunks packed – four of which contained only souvenirs, which also overflowed into other trunks.[29]

The day of departure came all too soon. Mrs Carpenter recalled:

> The morning of October 9*th*, 1886 dawned bright and clear. The carriage was ordered half an hour in advance of the train, that Anandibai might see once more every home that had been open to her, and take a last look at that she called her own. The bright sun and the soft air were not too bright or soft for this parting hour. The motion of the cars made her uncomfortable and she leaned on my shoulder for support until we reached the carriage in New York. This took us to the 'Etruria'. She was

very weak, but sat firmly in her seat as we drove; looking almost as bright as the flowers she carried. She was glad to lie down as soon as we reached the steamer. Not for a moment did she give way. A struggle between her weak body and her strong soul had been going on for days.[30]

Anandibai and Gopalrao were accompanied to the steamer by the entire Carpenter family, Pandita Ramabai, and Mr Sathe.[31]

Notes

1 Bodley, p. ii. The details of the much-emphasised blood relationship between Anandibai and Ramabai remain unknown.
2 Dall, pp. 128–29.
3 Dall, p. 129.
4 *Letters and Correspondence of Pandita Ramabai*, p. 165.
5 Dall, pp. 130–31.
6 Ibid, p. 131.
7 Ibid, pp. 134–35.
8 Ibid, p. 164.
9 Ibid, pp. 135–36.
10 Ibid, pp. 148–49.
11 Ibid, pp. 149–50.
12 Ibid, p. 152.
13 Ibid, pp. 153–55.
14 Ibid, p. 161.
15 Ibid, pp. 161–62.
16 Ibid, p. 163. The patchwork quilt was brought to India with Anandibai's other possessions and later acquired by the Raja Kelkar Museum at Pune where it is currently exhibited.
17 Dall, p. 162.
18 Ibid.
19 Kanitkar, pp. 269–70.
20 Dall, pp. 158–59.
21 Ibid, pp. 159–61.
22 Kanitkar, p. 281, my translation.
23 Dall, pp. 164–65.
24 Ibid, p. 166.
25 Ibid, p. 171.
26 Ibid, pp. 167–68.
27 Ibid, pp. 171–72.
28 Cited in Ibid, p. 169.
29 Ibid.
30 Ibid, p. 170.
31 Ibid, pp. 170–71.

Part III

THE RETURN OF THE NATIVE

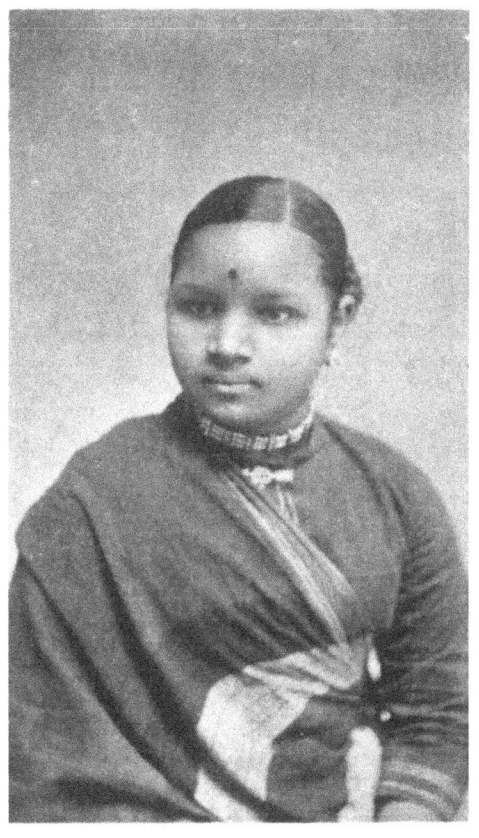

Figure PIII.1 Anandibai with her modified dress in the USA
Source: Photo courtesy Mr William J. Cobb

14

HOMEWARD BOUND

The Joshees' return journey was difficult, and was further aggravated by Anandibai's worsening health. Its eagerly awaited details were supplied to Mrs Carpenter by Gopalrao, who proved to be as regular a correspondent as Anandibai had been before being rendered incapable of putting pen to paper.[1]

11*th* Oct. 1886, on board the Etruria.

Two nights we have passed in this steamer. Today the sea is very rough, it shakes us very much. Dr Joshee is confined to her bed since we left the shore. She is not so much affected by cough as she was when in Roselle, but she is seasick – throws out everything she takes in. she is full of hopes. I have had a very bad cold and cough since I left New York. The Doctor and all other officers are very attentive. We get all we want, but we cannot eat . . .

12*th*. I could not write more yesterday, the steamer was so troublesome. Today also it is the same. Your niece asks me to tell you that she is still sick, though her cough does not disturb her so much. It is much better. I am sure it will leave her, if she keeps her chest and neck warm. . . .

I am not feeling well. Her sickness is coming to me. I have a sore throat and a cold in my head.

13*th*. Last night we spent in great distress of mind. Dr Joshee again caught cold in her chest, and the tickling of cough was so constant that we at once resorted to the severest dose of medicine. Brandy was given in hot and cold water, besides Dr Galt's medicine repeated after 10 minutes. The weather being so bad and rough we had to be rolling to and fro. Light went out. Dr Joshee inclined to . . . both upward and downward. I prayed to God for mercy. It was the severest trial I ever met with in my life. We were all the time joking and saying things, which made Dr Joshee so repentful? that she began to wish farewell to all. 'I am going now, my time has come. Send my respects to Aunt and several . . . India'. This was not all, but along with such repetitions, she shed tears profusely. I asked what was the matter? Why she was so frail? To which she replied, saying that she was trying to cry out these four days, but she could not do so while I was watching her so closely, but now I cannot refrain was her exclamation . . . I removed her this morning in order to ventilate her bed, but it was not five minutes before she wanted to be in bed again. The doctor came this morning, and gave her some sleeping medicine. She is better now. . . .

14*th*. We had a very bad storm last night. The steamer would have been smashed to pieces had it not been for her strength and bulk. The crew said they seldom experienced such bad weather in their trips. Dr Joshee is better today – slept all the time.

15*th*. Today it has been mild. Dr Joshee . . . seems sprightly and willing to go on deck, but the trouble we have in dressing her hair is another anxiety. I could not do it nicely. She therefore had to do it herself, which exhausted her so much, that all the vigour she showed vanished in the twinkling of an eye. . . . It is again supper time. Dr Joshee is resting well. I forgot to tell you the mischief Mr S – [*Sathe*] did, perhaps unknowingly. I had told him to take the valise in his hand when he went to New York, but he did not do it, in consequence of which, all the bottles contained therein were smashed to pieces; not only that, but Dr Joshee's night-gown and woollen dresses were soiled. There was one sweet-oil bottle and one other cod-liver oil. . . . [T]he room itself became unbearable. I am sorry things were so spoilt. The crackers Mr Carpenter gave us are gone. My papers and books suffered the same fate. . . . we shall reach Queenstown tomorrow.

London. Oct. 21*st*, 86. We arrived at Liverpool at 9 a.m. on the 17*th*, and stayed one night there. Instead of sailing yesterday, as already arranged, by the steamer Hergoda, we proceed today by the P. and O. Company's steamer Peshawar. I shall give particulars in my next . . .

Gibraltar, Oct. 26*th*, 86 – So far we have come. Nineteen days more, and then we come to the end of our journey. Dr Joshee is one day silver and one day gold. After trials and difficulties, both pecuniary and on account of race distinctions, we at last succeeded in securing a berth for Dr Joshee and a deck for myself. Dr Joshee was in good humour on the day we left London, was able to go on deck without assistance. I, being her native servant, had to be absent from her till I was sent for. Next day Dr Joshee went on deck, took her books and sat reading there. . . . now she is again confined to her bed, pains in her hands and feet, just as bad as it was when she returned home from Philadelphia. . . . Now I am again near her day and night, and she will be soon better. On this steamer we are obliged to put up with all sorts of inconveniences and social troubles. . . . It has been very smooth and calm on the sea since yesterday. In fact there was less botheration from water than there has been from men. You know I had $150 with me. I had to pay $100 additional for Dr Joshee. For myself, as her servant, I paid $100 only. The freight, board and lodging in London cost $60 for three days. Deduct your $150 from $260 expended by us. The surplus or deficiency is $110. Where did it come from in a country where we have had no friends? But 'God helps those who help themselves'. A strange lady unexpectedly came in, and seeing that we were in a fix, gave us a cheque for $90, and we owe Cook & Son $20. You may naturally be curious why we did not go by the steamer in which we had secured a berth for Dr Joshee. We were refused the passage at the 11*th* hour on account of our colour. There were two alternatives, either to wait for some time till we got a berth in some other steamer, or take the one just going. I preferred the latter course, however expensive and costly, that I might be free from blame in case of serious illness or otherwise. So we are home-bound. . . . I have sent some account to The Index of Boston. . . .

P.S. you must thank me for a letter herewith enclosed from Dr Joshee, the first of its kind since she left New York, 17 days ago. G.V.J.

Anandibai had written

I am not able to write a long letter, but I did want to say something to you about my health. I think I am a good deal stronger, though my cough is bad yet and my bronchitis somewhat worse. . . . I am getting over my seasickness, which has prevented me from getting proper nourishment or exercise. I am still in bed-have poultices on all day. The Doctor comes to see me twice daily. I am writing this in bed while lying down – shall write more next time.

With love to all. There has not been a day since the 9*th* when I did not miss your precious company.

Very affectionately,
Your niece, Anandibai Joshee

Here Mrs Carpenter adds: 'This I think was the last that she ever wrote to anybody'.

*

While in the United States, Gopalrao had obviously established good rapport with the *Index*, and also promised to write for them accounts of his travel home. The first of his letters, in which he at last got his longed-for opportunity to 'abuse the English' to his heart's content (while complimenting Americans to underscore the contrast) appeared on 18 November 1886 under the rubric 'A Hindoo's Opinion of England'. It had been written on 29 October and mailed *en route* to India.

His description of Liverpool was that '[h]alf the landing pier was filled with bare-footed [sic] boys and girls, the signs of the abject state of England. There were so many to see us off at New York, but none to receive us except the illegitimate issues of the English paupers'. What struck him next to the poverty of the people was the allegedly sub-standard police force. 'An American policeman is civil in disposition and majestic in appearance, but the English police is military in spirit and servile in behaviour; a cent or two easily buys one up; . . . the English police is a toy, and nothing more'. Next, the custom officers come in for criticism, for rigidly following the rules and lacking common sense in insisting on opening the Joshees' boxes instead of letting them go through to India. In two days in England Gopalrao noticed a meanness of spirit which he had not noticed in his eighteen months' stay in the United States. Their travel from Liverpool to London was accomplished by rail: The railway cars were almost empty, and people only travelled by third class, claims Gopalrao, 'in close compartments like prisoners' cells. The railway stations looked more like stables'. Gopalrao indicts everything English:

London water tasteless, air impure, horizon smoky, sky cloudy, outlook monotonous, street crowds melancholy and laden with cares; omnibuses dirty, no innovations in conveyances . . . Of all things, that which pained me most to look at is the miserable condition of the English women. I scarcely noticed a woman decently dressed in the streets of London; even the American factory girls are better dressed, as if they were of rank and position. . . . Nowhere in Europe, except England and Germany, are there so many thousands of rude and illiterate people. . . . the rural population of India may be illiterate as far as reading and writing are concerned, but their moral and ethical education is not far from completion.

Gopalrao's next letter published in the *Index* (23 December 1886), was written on 31 October and mailed from Port Said, and was not only inordinately long but also far more vituperative on account of the indignities which the Joshees suffered in London. For their onward journey to India, a berth had been booked for the ailing Anandibai (whose passage was paid for by Kolhapur State) while Gopalrao was to travel as a deck passenger. This berth was now refused to her for reasons of racial discrimination, claimed Gopalrao in the letter captioned 'An Indignant Letter from a Hindu Brahmin'.

A buoyant, burlesque [sic], young looking English cur [at Cook & Son's office] told me that a berth was reserved, but he did not know it was for a Hindu lady. The company and the agents do not book any Hindu passengers because of the avowed reluctance of the white passengers to travel with a Hindu in their company. . . . [A]s the passage money was not paid, he would not grant a ticket for the Hindu lady.

The Joshees then had a visit from some American acquaintances – Mr and Mrs Pattison – then in England, who were upset at this unnecessary problem and who gave Gopalrao 'a cheque for eighty or ninety pounds'. (In his letter to Mrs Carpenter, he had mentioned a cheque for ninety dollars.) Finally, Anandibai's first class passage was booked, but a 'white, soldierly fellow', probably a purser, tried to evict her, again on racial grounds. Gopalrao claimed that during her stay in the United States, Anandibai had had no experience of the 'animosity between the black and white races' of the kind 'fostered by the English'; 'she was respectfully treated as a lady'. The only country that could bring the English to their senses was Russia, thought Gopalrao – which explains his attraction for that country.

Anandibai was not visited by the doctor or the stewardess until expressly sent for – in contrast to the doctor on the New York–Liverpool steamer – and the stewardess took her for a servant or a child's *ayah*. Fellow passengers took no notice of her. Gopalrao himself was told by the purser that he had nowhere to sit during the day or sleep at night, except on deck in severe cold: 'I have travelled far and wide, but never saw elsewhere such heartless, brutal mortals as the English are today in India'. The crowning insult was that no food suitable for vegetarians was made available to Anandibai. When she declined meat dishes, explaining that she abstained from animal food, she was promptly offered beef tea. Starvation was the result.[2]

This letter from the *Index* stirred up a hornet's nest, especially in England, as he had obviously anticipated. Both parties to the incident were ardently championed: the steamship company by Mrs Dall among others, and Gopalrao unexpectedly by Pandita Ramabai. In her letter to Miss Beale, principal of Cheltenham College, where she had received teacher training, she was able to corroborate Gopalrao's story, except that the amount of money lent by Mr Pattison was eighteen pounds, not eighty (which he later paid back).

*

The Joshees' onward voyage continued more smoothly, as Gopalrao reported to Mrs Carpenter:

> Port Said, 3*rd* November 1886. S.S. Peshawar.
> My dear Madam,
> We are all safe at Port Said. We will enter the Suez Canal today. Now 12 days to reach native land. Dr Joshee is full of hopes. She feels better as she nears her country. What does she want to do on landing? I answer for her. She wants to eat her food. She daily mentions thousand and one things that she likes to eat. . . . It is bright now. We had very stormy weather. Dr Joshee does not feel like lifting up her head.
> Aden, *en route* to India; 9*th* November 1886. I post this at Aden. Today is one month since we have been separated from you. On our way there have been several ups and downs. In [sic] the Red Sea, these three days, it has been intensely warm. We were perspiring day and night. Dr Joshee had to do away with her flannel wrappers. Her tickling cough still disturbs her. It has not abated in the least. Her low state of health precludes taking any nourishment. She brings out everything she eats. The Surgeon on board recommended champagne, brandy, claret and whisky. She drank more of them in these 15 days, than she did in America in 3 years.

Here Mrs Carpenter comments, 'Dr Joshee never took stimulants except for medicine, and never for that, if she thought it avoidable'.

Gopalrao continues:

> I am almost sure drinking kept down her temperature too low. She had no taste for anything. You know how difficult it is to get what she likes. On the 'Etruria' we were specially cared for in consequence of Mr Carpenter's letter to the agent. But on this steamer, everything we get is a favour. From today I have suggested that she take no more stimulants, but let nature cure her. She will be now in her own country. It would therefore be wise to discontinue all European medicines and live on [a] plain simple diet. But she is a doctor now and will not, I am afraid, heed my suggestion. One more happy news for you. On board the steamer we were regularly persecuted; at the same time, someone who came to know of our being refused another steamer sent word to us that if we needed any money he would be very glad to lend and receive it back at our convenience, say 100 years hence. I have not personally seen him, nor do I know which of the passengers is our benefactor. To make the story short, you come across good souls if you travel as I have always done, but money in pockets makes you distrust everybody.

Perhaps this was Gopalrao's way of restoring the gender balance: After having been the unremarkable, unemployed, and eccentric husband of a much lionised Indian woman doctor, he was now once again the lord and master who could command obedience from his doctor-wife to his prescription that 'all European medicines' should be discontinued out of respect for Indian customs. After three years of intense medical training, Anandibai was to be reduced to the average submissive wife whose hard-earned expertise could be overruled at will by her husband who had no claim to medical knowledge – in a matter of her own life and death.

Notes

1 Gopalrao's letters were copied out by Mrs Carpenter in her own handwriting.
2 The letter is partly reproduced by Dall, p. 173.

15

THE LAST FLICKER

When she landed at Mumbai early in the morning of 16 November 1886, Anandibai had reverted to her earlier Maharashtrian persona – a black nine-yard sari, *khun* blouse, nose-ring and ear studs, the only 'modern touch' being shoes and stockings.[1] This was to be immortalised as much – or more than – her travel abroad and her medical degree. The Joshees were welcomed by a group of Gopalrao's friends amid a shower of flowers, and then accompanied to their destination. Seeking to make up for Mumbai's allegedly disappointing, low-key reception, *The Mahratta* (21 November 1886) extended an enthusiastic welcome on behalf of Pune, Maharashtra's cultural heartland:

> We bid a hearty welcome to Mr Gopalrao Joshi [sic] and his wife Dr Anandibai Joshee, who returned to India by the last Mail Steamer. The plucky pair has laid all India under deep obligation by the noble example set by it of self-help, great moral courage, perseverance and indomitable will to overcome every difficulty . . . Happy it is that the worthy husband and wife have conquered all these difficulties and come back to India again with Western culture but without a taint of Western vice. Mrs Joshee has preserved her Hindu habits and customs and that too at no small personal inconvenience . . . We hope Poona society – all sections of Poona society – the orthodox people as well as reformers, will duly appreciate the worth of Mrs Anandibai's heroic act and will give her a sincere and cordial welcome. It is a pity that the Bombay people did not do anything to show to the young lady how they appreciate the valuable example set by her.

The paper compared this unfavourably with the enthusiastic farewell given to Pandita Ramabai at her departure for England three years earlier. Three issues emerged prominently in the article and were to be echoed over the decade to form a sharply etched image of Anandibai: her (and by extension Gopalrao's) courage, perseverance, intellectual effort, and achievement; her traditional dress, diet, and behaviour; and her moral superiority to Pandita Ramabai. A fourth issue that also emerged in other papers – as for example in *Subodha Patrika* cited below – was the attribution of credit for Anandibai's achievement to Gopalrao.

Although faulted by *The Mahratta*, the citizens of Mumbai, held to be liberal in contrast to the generally conservative Poonaites, were not really backward in their attentions. *Subodha Patrika*, the organ of Mumbai's Prarthana Samaj, had expressed its admiration for the Joshees also on 21 November:

> We are very happy to report that our compatriot and friend Mr Gopalrao Joshee has returned, after achieving all his aims, having given his wife Dr Mrs Anandibai an excellent English education and having succeeded in getting her the medical degree of MD in America . . . We were greatly pleased to see that there was no ostentation and display, no inflated importance for their American travel, no arrogance; and everything was simple![2]

The installation of Anandibai's image as a passive creation of Gopalrao's had already started.

The wonder woman, India's first woman doctor, could still be reclaimed primarily as a daughter of Maharashtra on the strength of her traditional dress alone. It was hardly surprising that, having constructed women as the repositories of culture and carriers of tradition, mainstream society willingly freed men from both responsibilities. Hardly a comment was made about Gopalrao's dress or diet during his two and a half years' absence from India.[3]

Only *Kesari* (23 November 1886) struck an additional and socially conscious note in welcoming the Joshees:

> Our country has a prejudice against female education, our women are extraordinarily modest and dislike stepping out of the home to undertake brave deeds; even our men fear travel and sea voyage. In view of all this and after considering the obstacles probably faced by Mr Gopalrao with regard to finances and public opinion, one cannot bestow sufficient praise on his determination to give his wife a useful education in the interests of national service, and on Mrs Anandibai's

courage, resolution and hard work in acting in deferential obedience to her husband's command.

The assumption that the radical idea of Anandibai's medical education was Gopalrao's and that Anandibai merely acquiesced in his plans for her was already deep-rooted. That she could think for herself or had a voice in sculpting her future did not occur to her contemporaries: 'The example set by Mr Gopalrao and Anandibai is amazing and worthy of emulation. We should make arrangements to ensure that the knowledge acquired by Mrs Anandibai is utilised not in the service of a Native State, but in the permanent interests of the women here'.

*

Anandibai herself was to prove her traditional Maharashtrian credentials in more concrete terms. On their arrival in Mumbai, the Joshees stayed with her maternal aunt's son. The very same day, they received news of this aunt's death. Greatly grieved, Anandibai observed the custom of having a ritual bath, pouring water over her head, against everybody's advice. It was a relatively cool November day and she ran a fever that evening which considerably aggravated her condition. Nor did the damp and overcrowded accommodation provide much comfort.[4]

Soon the Joshees moved to the house of the famous Gujarati philanthropist Seth Madhavdas Raghunathdas Kapadia, who welcomed them warmly in Mumbai's true cosmopolitan spirit. There was a constant stream of visitors wishing to converse with the celebrity; and the exhausted Anandibai denied nobody.[5]

Gopalrao wrote his first letter to Mrs Carpenter on 25 November; his earlier note had not reached her:

> The first two days Dr Joshee was lively and spirited, but the energy soon vanished, and she was again confined to her bed with increased cough and fever. Today [the] cough is entirely gone and [the] fever abated, but weakness has taken possession of her. Her mother, younger sister and brother, and grandmother have come down to see her, but we have not yet been able to give her that kind of food which would be relished by her. Although her mother and grandmother are here, yet they have not got all the materials to prepare choice dishes. We are living in a house where people, nay, the host and hostess are too good-natured – as devoted as our own relatives would be, but their diet does not exactly suit our tastes, hence the

inconvenience. You will understand how difficult it is for us to get on in our own country, so divided we are in every respect.

Mrs Carpenter's comment on the last statement was 'this reminds me of what Dr Joshee once wrote of the great difference of people living at a short distance in India'.

Anandibai was obviously too ill to think of joining her duties at Kolhapur immediately and was granted leave for a few days; she seemed confident of her eventual recovery. The immediate plans remained uncertain; an extended stay in Mumbai involved the acute problem of accommodation. The Joshees' perpetual moves sound extremely exhausting; there was obviously no clear plan and any future move probably hinged on the latest and the most convincing medical opinion. (One assumes that Anandibai's eleven trunks of baggage went with them.) They went into rented rooms in Girgaum. Many of Anandibai's close relatives had come to be with her. Medical opinion was sought, and diagnoses varied from acute exhaustion to something far more serious, and treatment changed accordingly.[6] After a few days, the family moved again, but only temporarily. Gopalrao informed Mrs Carpenter on 3 December:

> We are still in Bombay. It is so uncertain as to what should be done next. Dr Joshee's sickness is a matter of great concern with our people who all long for her speedy recovery. God may bless these wishes and send relief immediately.
>
> We have been removing from house to house. Today we are in a third place, and a fourth is not far distant. You know how troublesome it is for a sick person to be going about, but we can't help it. The place we first went to was unfurnished and newly built; consequently very damp. The next one was comfortable but temporary. It was given us for a week or so but we continued in it 16 days. Yesterday afternoon and morning Dr Joshee was bright and lively, but in the evening exhaustion, brought about by removal, reacted upon her. . . . Dr Joshee asks me to request you to write to 4 medical journals, as she would like to subscribe for them: 1) Journal of Obstetrics & Surgery, 2) New York Record, 3) Philadelphia Medical World, 4) London Lancet. Subscription will be sent when she joins the appointment at Kolhapur. I have written this much at her request, that you may see that she has still the same energy and ambition to be useful to her people. . . . my mind is heavily laden with care. There are so many anxieties. The first and foremost is that of

Dr Joshee – how she will recover. I sometimes grow hopeless, sometimes hopeful. There is my mother anxiously waiting [at Sangamner] for money for sundry expenses. Here we have no friends at our disposal. But such is life and so we are.

Anandibai's progress was being monitored at Pune. *Kesari* (7 December 1886) reported that 'Dr Anandibai Joshee has been unwell since her arrival at Mumbai. She is under treatment'.

After about three weeks in Mumbai, the diagnosis of consumption seems to have been confirmed; doctors recommended the dry climate of the hills and suggested Pune. This suited Gopalrao's plan to try the Ayurvedic treatment of the famous *Vaidya*, or indigenous physician, Mr Mehendale. This was possibly Gopalrao's final attempt to prove the superiority of Indian medicine over Western. The family rushed to Pune directly, alarmed by Anandibai's rapidly declining health.[7] Gopalrao wrote to Mrs Carpenter from Mumbai on 9 December:

I drop you a word in haste. We leave for Poona today. The climate of Bombay is very depressing, and Dr Joshee wishes to go to Poona since we arrived here, but the doctors who attended upon, or examined her case, pronounced that it was not safe for her to go up-country, as sea breezes are more favourable to her complaint. But this decision had a very bad effect on her constitution. She lost more flesh in India than she did in America or on her voyage. We, however, found one eminent doctor among Europeans who recommended up-country climate, as he said that it is more bracing than sea climate. We therefore proceed to Poona. I have a mind to place her entirely under native treatment, as Western one is very trying in delicate cases. Dr Joshee is merely a skeleton of bones and skin, and the case is pronounced to be very serious. I have still great hopes. Man is not able to say with certainty what God proposes to do. I am so unsettled in my plans and ways and means, that I hardly find time to write as I did on board the steamer. Here people flock in all the time, and I have to attend to them. Dr Joshee is now a national centre. Whole India is sorry for her illness. She is full of hope as she always has been. . . . we reach Poona at 7 p.m.

*

On 9 December the whole family went to Pune by the two o'clock train, Anandibai and her mother travelling first class, and the rest (her sister, brother, and Gopalrao himself), third class.[8] A public welcome awaited Anandibai at Pune, if not in person, at least through newspapers. The *Mahratta* (12 December 1886) wrote:

> We welcome Dr Anandi Bai Joshi [sic] back to Poona. Unfortunately, since her arrival in Bombay, she has been confined to her bed and comes up here for [a] change, Poona being her birth-place. The Poonaites had, therefore, to forgo the pleasure of receiving her as she deserves at this time. Dr Joshee was suffering [from] cough before she left America, and the sea-journey has told upon her health considerably. She is now suffering from high fever and it is said that the cough has nearly affected her lungs. We earnestly hope that the Poona climate restores her to health soon and that the fruits of her enterprise [will] be soon made available to the public.

The family's disorganised schedule continued also at Pune. The first accommodation had to be changed within a week for reasons of convenience and the family was invited by Rao Bahadur Vishnu Moreshwar Bhide to his mansion. It was a comfortable stay. Bhide placed his carriage at their disposal, and Gopalrao forced Anandibai to drive out with him every evening even though she could barely walk to the carriage.[9] His autocratic behaviour, ostensibly for her own good, must have proved counter-productive on many occasions. She continued to obey him without demur, as always.

Immediately on reaching Pune, Gopalrao contacted Bapusaheb Mehendale, the famous *Vaidya*, through friends. But he refused to treat Anandibai. Several eminent people of the city tried to persuade him, and Anandibai added a request of her own; but he was adamant, on the ostensible grounds that Anandibai was 'learned in foreign medical knowledge' and could not be treated by a person of his 'inferior qualifications'. The conflations of acute rivalry between the two medical systems and the patriarchal resentment for a woman's obtaining a medical degree were too strong to unbend him. Another *Vaidya* of repute was then approached, this time with greater success.[10] It may be added, however, that thus far, Ayurvedic treatment had not succeeded in curing tuberculosis.

On 16 December Gopalrao wrote to Mrs Carpenter:

> Today I write from the place where Dr Joshee was born. This city is high land. Bombay is low. When we ascended the summits of the mountains and Dr Joshee breathed cool breezes from the land, she felt refreshed and lively. Three consecutive

days her cough abated considerably without any medicine, so that climatic changes influence her very favourably. But as she is sickly and weak in constitution, it was natural for us to consult doctors again for treating her. One doctor in whom we have full confidence was sent for, and prescribed mild native medicine, but unfortunately instead of improvement, collapse was the result. Dr Joshee felt intensely excited, mouth became tasteless, and appetite slackened again, cough excessively set in, and she refused to taste the same medicine. The Bombay doctors, both native and European, have considered the case beyond cure, so that I could not do better than place her under native treatment. But here also we have consulted one who has studied English works. . . .

Her mother, grandmother, elder and younger sisters and brother, as well as aunts and cousins are here. It is a case of consumption. . . . she was always feverish even before she left India. . . . most of the Poona people have been praying for her recovery. . . . I am sure she needs Homeopathic treatment. That will give her relief. . . . [and] she will not find it so troublesome as swallowing large doses. Last night we all were awake, the cough was so troublesome. People call on us at all hours, and it is so unpleasant to refuse admittance. Sometimes ladies call, some out of curiosity, some out of anxiety and sympathy. Those who would scarcely slip out come to see her, some good orthodox and superstitious – all forgetting that we had been to America. It is a novel sight, most interesting to meditate upon. But Dr Joshee's illness is the concern for all. Do pray for her recovery. Superstition has not left us. [We perform rituals.] The Brahmins come every day and apply some ashes to Dr Joshee's forehead. She then puts a bit in her mouth. . . . Dr Joshee is sitting on the couch, her fingers turning on her eyelids, all happy and in good humour; sometimes disturbed by coughs. She heartily joins with me in saying that we wish you all a happy Christmas and New Year.

In late December the Joshees were asked to make alternative arrangements for their accommodation, and moved again. On Anandibai's health front, the pendulum continued to swing from hope to despair. Gopalrao's letter to Mrs Carpenter on 23 December said

these three days Dr Joshee has been feeling pretty well. She scoffs at the idea of consumption, which all the doctors say she is suffering from. Hindu doctors have a different opinion. They say it is simple bronchitis and nothing [more]. Now she is under treatment of her own relative, the brother of her grand-mother [Balshastri Mate]. . . . some of the local papers have devoted columns to Dr Joshee's sympathy. . . . Dr Joshee has read your letters over and over again. It has proved a tonic to her in her sickness. A kind and encouraging word from you is worth millions. I will write to you, and you reply to her, so that she will think of it as her own [letter]. . . . She has a strong individuality.

Gopalrao's claims about the extent of public interest in and newspa-per reports on Anandibai were exaggerated. Of the two papers he was most closely associated with, the *Mahratta* made no mention of her at this time, and *Kesari* (28 December) gave only a brief notice:

Dr Mrs Anandibai has been unwell and has come here for a change of weather, as the readers know. We understand that the Poona climate has improved her health considerably and that the physicians expect her health to be completely restored in two or three months.[11]

On 6 January, Gopalrao reported to Mrs Carpenter that 'Dr Joshee shows some signs of improvement. She is still under native treatment'. On 1 January he added: '*Your letter came just in time to cheer up your niece. She has not been feeling so brisk and lively the last week. Her medi-cine has changed*'.

Predictably Anandibai's improvement was short-lived. One osten-sible reason, advanced by Gopalrao, was that she was unable to fol-low the strict diet mandated by Ayurvedic remedies: Her mother had indulged her with her favourite Maharashtrian dishes, which she had craved for during the previous three years, against the physician's orders. On the other hand, Gopalrao himself contributed in no small measure to the aggravation of her condition. The latest Ayurvedic remedy was a boiled mixture of several herbs to be taken daily for seven days. One of the herbs was *adulsa*, which alleviated cough. Seven leaves daily were to be added to the boiled mixture during the first week, fourteen during the second week, and twenty-one during the third. In his attempt to expedite her recovery, he increased the dosage to fourteen leaves on the second day, and then twenty-one, overriding her protests. The result, as she had feared, was diarrhoea which caused a considerable setback.[12]

Anandibai was in agony most of the time, but bore it without a grimace or a groan. She tried to receive all visitors; if she appeared unwilling when a particularly garrulous visitor was announced, Gopalrao immediately reprimanded her for her conceit so that she had to give in. Her obedience to him never wavered. Among the sisters were Anandibai's two married sisters who lived in Pune; they could come only late in the evening and sat talking into the night. Whatever sleep Anandibai could snatch was disturbed by cough or nightmares centering usually on the lost job at the Kolhapur hospital: In her dreams she saw her examination of the patients interrupted by missionary ladies who propagated the Bible, the scene turning into manifest rivalry and conflict.[13]

The Joshee's situation was aggravated by depleted funds. Gopalrao had no job. Anandibai was initially technically on leave at half-pay from her position at the Kolhapur hospital, but her application for an extension of leave was refused at this time, automatically terminating her contract with Kolhapur State. She accepted the situation with her usual philosophical calm. Financial help, however, came from unexpected quarters. A wealthy and eminent resident of Pune, aware of the Joshees' financial straits but unwilling to help himself, informed Lady Reay, wife of the Governor of the Bombay Presidency. She, with a lady friend, sent Anandibai Rs 100. A small contribution also came from the editors of *Kesari* and the *Mahratta*.

The routine Ayurvedic medicines had failed to provide relief. Now the last and most desperate remedy was to be tried, and Anandibai was seemingly pressured to consent. As Gopalrao wrote on 10 February 1887:

> I have to repeat the same sad story, that my wife is still confined to her bed. She has no strength to stand or sit right. Professional men pronounce the case to be hopeless, but I have a firm belief that it is not so. There is yet room to recover, but where is that doctor, no one knows. Today she is convalescent and tomorrow again worse, so that I am at a loss to convey any correct information to my American well-wishers and sympathizers. When we came to Poona, we had put up with a gentleman who disinterestedly placed at our disposal his well-furnished hall and made us as comfortable as we could desire under the circumstances. But now we are in another place of our own – that is a hired one.

One wonders whether Gopalrao was by this time so used to being looked after in comfort by philanthropists in India (as he had been in the United States), for his wife's sake, that he resented having to manage on his own, especially now that he was not employed.

> [The] day before yesterday we were all afraid of meeting the worst possible. But doctors were sent for at midnight, and they gave temporary relief. Yesterday we tried another doctor of good repute, who has specific remedies on consumption. But the administration of them was a difficult job. The medicine was to be given on one condition, that is to say, no water would be given to the patient for 7 days. She must drink milk whenever she should feel thirsty. We prevailed upon her to take that medicine, and she did take [it], but before 12 hours were over, she was exceedingly thirsty, and longed and begged for water, but we could not yield to her importunities. At last after 24 hours we gave her water, but the medicine seemed to be a real specific on the disease. I am sorry that Dr Joshee should not recover yet, but His will be done.

The abruptly terminated treatment reduced Anandibai to such weakness that she was unable to even lift her hand.

It was in this state that Anandibai was moved to her maternal granduncle's mansion – the very mansion where she was born less than twenty-two years earlier. This gentleman, Balshastri Mate, had treated her sporadically, even as Gopalrao kept on trying out different physicians. But now the situation deteriorated rapidly. On Friday, 25 February, Gopalrao stayed by her bedside the whole day, perhaps sensing that it was to be his last day with her.[14]

On 28 February, Gopalrao wrote in agony to Mrs Carpenter:

> My dear aunt,
> I do not know how I should address you, but I am helpless today. There was only one who could address you thus, but God has deprived you and me of that dear charming soul, the fortress of courage, patience and forbearance. Dr Joshee, where is she now? Left this world for good on Saturday the 26th at about midnight . . . Friday last I was in attendance whole night. No posture was comfortable to her. I was all the time shifting her from one side to another. The breathing was so loud that I feared that it would immediately burst out the whole system, so that the whole night passed in restlessness and painfulness. In the morning, that is on Saturday, the whole case was placed

before her doctor. He advised me to give her two grams of opium. I did so. It gave her relief. . . . the opium stopped the coughing. . . . but we did not know the worst was in store for us to narrate. We entertained her in the afternoon so that she passed the day in apparent ease. The breathing was not so hard, but there was, as usual, [a] chill followed by strong fever. These 20 days she has been extremely weak, having no strength to move her head. Oh Fate! What is thy work on earth? Why didst thou bother this poor innocent soul?

At about 8 p.m. I raised her to a sitting posture, making myself a pillow for her to lean against. Her mother was serving her. Dr Joshee had [an] appetite, but no sooner was food put into her mouth than vomiting sensations set in. I rebuked her mother for not preparing things nicely and tastefully [sic], but my poor wife did not like that remark. She said it was not the food she did not like, but something was the matter with her. I gave her to drink milk which she did retain, and then laid her down. She was apparently comfortable, not so disturbed as she had been for the past few days. Her feet were swollen. There was swelling on her face also. At about 10 o'clock I gave her a second dose of medicine, and then went to bed. I was fast asleep when she breathed her last. Her mother was, however, by her side. Poor Anandibai called 'mother' three times, and ceased to breathe. By the time her mother takes her up to her breast, pulsation stopped. There was jerking in her hands and throat, and strong motions in her sides. Her mother cried loudly, 'Gone! Gone!!' her grandmother and aunt went right there. They went to her bed, simply to return to awaken me, her brother and the doctor in attendance, in whose house we have returned these 12 days. I was always up at first call, but that night twenty howling sounds were not enough to break my sleep. Presence of mind was lost, and I was running like a madman just to think what to do next. The doctor came to her bed and examined her pulse. We poured some strong medicine into her mouth by forcibly opening her jaws. . . .

Since the administration of the milk medicine, of which I had given you some particulars in my last, she lost all vitality. I have had no time to drop you a line these two weeks. One mail day passed away without my knowledge. We were in constant fear of meeting the <u>inevitable</u>; some relief was felt afterward, and we hoped for better, but another fit came which necessitated our seeking another doctor, though doctors have been her curse, and she succumbed to her own hobby. We again removed to her relative, who, if you remember, I told you was first attending upon her. He is her grandmother's own brother. Dr Joshee was born in his house, and would perhaps recover there. That was our reason. Another was that he being very old, about 75, could attend to her at will. We therefore begged him to admit her into his house, to which he readily assented, so that we gladly moved. But the disease was so powerful, that he did not know how to check it. Her system was very much heated by former treatment. He cooled it down, and she passed the day quite comfortably. But the change from extreme heat to extreme cold produced diarrhoea. We went to check it and introduced wind in her stomach; consequently her legs and feet were swollen. Her pains were unspeakable, but Dr Joshee never indicated any anxieties on her countenance, or in her speaking, always ready to cheer up her surroundings. She several times expressed that she suppressed her pangs, that others might not suffer from her expositions. How brave and thoughtful!!! She was grave, gentle and meditative to the extreme. She never showed any childish distemper in her actions, no, never; she was deeply conscious that it was her duty to please the old folks.

She grew exceedingly religious. A touch from an outcast or a Christian was pollution. Do you believe me? It was so. She invariably ordered her waterpots to be removed if any European lady approached her. Nay, even her own maidservant need not put her feet upon the carpet which connected with her bedstead. I argued and showed the foolishness of such thoughts being entertained by one who had spent some years in America. Her plea was that her grandmother and widowed sister and mother have an abhorrence of such uncleanliness and she must try to please them. In one sense it was very considerate. Properly speaking, we ought to have been treated as regular outcasts, and our shadows shunned. But our people were very tolerant. Not a soul who knew us abstained from coming and paying us a visit – old and young, orthodox and other wise, all obliged us by conferring friendly visits. She never felt that she was treated otherwise than her connection with all sorts demanded. In that she was fortunate. Two or three days before her departure to the spirit world she had the satisfaction of performing the ceremony 'Pacification of Waters'. Brahmins were seated for dinner, and the old doctor sent for me, that I might sprinkle water on the banana leaves on which all the eatables were served. . . . if they had treated me as an outcast, they would not have allowed me to do so. But no, it was all right; and all good. I wished she had lived longer. As regards our people, all that we prophesied or predicted came to pass. There has been no opposition to us. Even the reformers were astonished as to how we were received and treated as friends in the most orthodox families. But such is the irony of fate. We conquered all opposition, all obstacles, but death. Destiny and Fate were insurmountable.

Gopalrao's fear about being ostracised for their foreign travel was not baseless.

Anandibai's body was bathed and dressed in her finery as befitted a married woman, and a photo was taken. Although time was short, a number of mourners came to the house and joined the funeral procession to the cremation ground. As Gopalrao wrote:

Here too our people are very kind. Even for rich families, if excommunicated, [pall] bearers are hard to get, but we had enough and to spare. Another difficulty was whether Brahmins could be had for funeral rites. I am glad to tell you all passed happily so far as external appearances were concerned. We gave her a religious fire.[15] There was a goodly crowd. People had no notice, nor could we keep the body longer. That warmness vanished, and the body became cold and changed. I now understand why death is said to be cold. I never before accompanied any one to the burning ground, and saw fire set to the pile of wood and cow-dung cakes.

The harsher reality of death finally caught up with Gopalrao at the age of forty, having so far been protected from it in spite of having lost his first wife and his father.

After Anandibai's body was placed on the funeral pyre, Mr V. M. Ranade made a speech in her honour, bemoaning the death of this intellectual, self-sacrificing soul at the age of twenty-one years and eleven months, 'on the threshold of the work for which she was so well equipped!'[16]

Mrs Carpenter notes:

In a subsequent letter Mr Joshee mentions that he had to perform funeral ceremonies up to 13 days.

Dr Joshee was in India 3 months and 10 days.

She was cremated on Saturday at 11 a.m.

In Mrs Carpenter's handwriting appear the following lines, originally either hers or Gopalrao's:

Alas! What sorrow is ours, who knew and loved her? The inevitable is upon us, and with a faith in God who doeth all things well let us bear this dispensation with hearts turned toward Him, believing that there is some wise providence in the early departure of this noble and beloved soul.

Anandibai's funeral photo was sent to America, and in Dr Bodley's words:

The pathos of that lifeless form is indescribable. The last of several pictures, taken during the brief public career of the little reformer, it is the most eloquent of them all. The mute lips and the face, wan and wasted and prematurely aged in the fierce battle with sorrow and pain, alike convey to her American friends the message, not to be forgotten: 'I have done all that I could do'.

Notes

1 Kanitkar, p. 282.
2 Cited in ibid, p. 283, my translation.
3 Incidentally the *Mahratta*'s (5 December 1886) words are quite revealing. In its report on Dr R.G. Bhandarkar's return from his visit to Europe at about the same time: 'Dr Bhandarkar had decided on keeping his Indian dress while in Europe, viz., his turban, his usual Bombay angarakha [traditional coat tied across the chest with strings] and trousers. People in England easily recognised him as an Indian in this dress'. A Europeanised dress with the token turban was enough to establish a man's Indianness abroad; for a woman such compromises were unthought of.
4 Kanitkar, p. 286.
5 Ibid.
6 Ibid.
7 Ibid, p. 289.
8 Ibid.
9 Ibid, p. 290.
10 Ibid.
11 My translation.
12 Kanitkar, p. 293.
13 Ibid, p. 295
14 Ibid, p. 296.
15 That is, cremation with all proper rites. These would be denied to an excommunicated person.
16 Cited in Dall, p. 186.

16

A DEATH MOURNED
AND LIVES RESUMED

Anandibai 'ceased upon the midnight', though perhaps not without pain, on Saturday, 26 February 1887.[1] She was cremated the following morning. The first newspaper to report the event was the weekly *Kesari*, published on Tuesdays.[2] *Kesari*'s short note (1 March 1887) said

> Mrs Anandibai has left us for her heavenly abode. But the example set by her will not fail to produce results. It is astonishing that a woman, and that too a woman of the Brahmin caste, should display such adventurousness, unceasing toil, disregard of rewards, intense desire for service to the nation, firm resolution, courage in the face of terrible calamities, etc. which are rarely found outside the male sex. We should erect a memorial as a testimony and permanent commemoration of such wonderful qualities; otherwise we will not be free of the debt in which Dr Anandibai has placed us. In our opinion, an excellent memorial will be the creation of a scheme by which another woman of her status will be enabled to follow the example set by this extraordinary lady.[3]

A comprehensive tribute was paid in an editorial in the same issue, which captured the essence of Anandibai's achievement, emphasising the hardships she had encountered and which would daunt a man in spite of his more privileged social location. This was Agarkar's own personal, emotional statement drawing Gopalrao into its orbit of sympathy as a partner in Anandibai's life and deeds.[4] Under the caption 'The Late Dr Mrs Anandibai Joshee', it says:

> There are those the country or a society owes a debt of gratitude for their physical prowess, intellectual strength, or altruism; and appropriately enough, the grateful people and historians

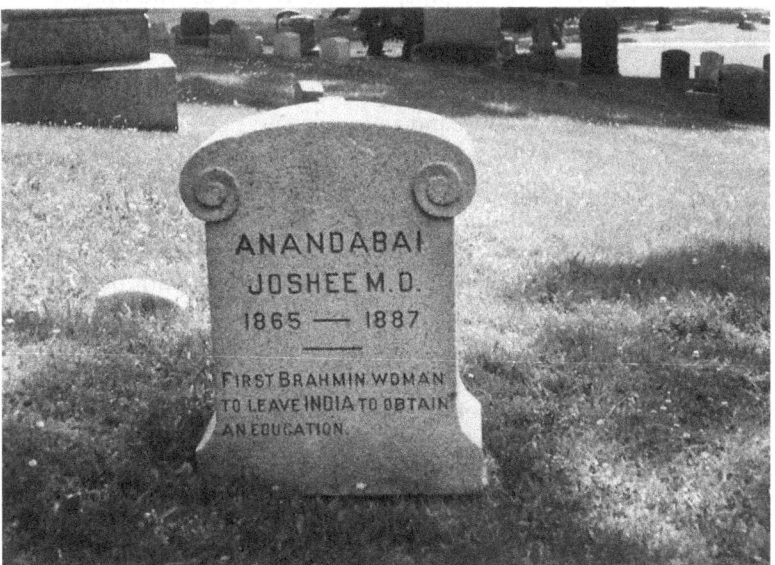

Figure 16.1 A closer view of Anandibai's grave-marker, summer 2004
Source: Photograph by the author

lovingly sing their praises and, through their stories, imprint an indelible image of virtue on the minds of young men and women. . . . The beliefs regarding women, deeply entrenched in this country for centuries, are that a woman is the shadow of a man, that her reason for existence is to spend her life in his service, that she is strictly forbidden to speak a few words freely even with her husband's friends, and that the ultimate limit of her achievements is the service of her elders, nuture of children, and domestic tasks. But can you, Readers, imagine anything more praiseworthy in a woman's achievement than that a married woman of this country should study a difficult foreign language like English at her husband's desire; that she should be ready to undertake a long sea voyage in the prime of her youth, without adequate financial support and by relying on men and women of a different religion; that she should obtain a university degree in a foreign continent after studying in a foreign language day and night for three or four years; and that, clearing all obstacles courageously, she should return to her home country with a heart filled with joy and anticipation at the prospect of carrying on the original purpose?

Here Agarkar also falls into the popular trap of casting Anandibai as a creation of her visionary husband and undercuts her agency. In that day and age it was either not possible to visualise or prudent not to mention a woman's independent thinking. Consequently, all subsequent obituaries offered credit for Anandibai's achievment to Gopalrao, and underscored her obedience to him, as well as qualities like perseverance, hard work, and intense desire to help Indian women with health care. Agarkar goes on to describe the harm caused to national reform by the sudden death of 'an invaluable person like Anandibai', and commiserates with Gopalrao, calling her his sister.

The following day, another Pune weekly, *Dnyana Chakshu* (2 March 1887), published its obituary, which was later translated by Pandita Ramabai for her American friends:

> Although Anandibai was so young, her preseverance, undaunted courage, and devotion to her husband were unparalleled. We think it will be long before we shall again see a woman like her in this country. We do not hesitate to say that Dr Joshee is worthy of a high place on the roll of historic women who have striven to serve and to elevate their native land. . . . the education she had received had greatly heightened her nature and ennobled her mind. Although she suffered more than words can express, from her mortal disease, phthisis [consumption], not a word of either complaint or impatience escaped her lips at any time.[5]

The paper valorised her silent suffering, even when she was reduced to skin and bones, and her appearance shocked and pained all visitors, and it described her cremation.

The reports in Mumbai papers were naturally delayed by a few days. The conservative *Native Opinion* (6 March 1889) published a short note in its English section. While deeply regretting Anandibai's death the note was generally critical in tone, and, held up her fate as a deterrent example of the disastrous results of a foreign education for Indian women:

> Being no admirers of entrusting the education of our women to stangers in strange lands, we may not be wrong in looking upon this sad event as one cumulative fatal result of foreign residence and its attendant wants, discomforts, and hard study.

However, there was one thing in her that deserves our admiration; her courage and strong desire to learn a science wherewith to be useful to the female portion of her own countrymen in India.

The same issue published a brief news item in the Marathi section, in which her stay in America was held responsible for her death: 'her diet in that country, which was not nutritious enough, led to the disease which ultimately resulted in her death'. Gopalrao emerged as the self-sacrificing sufferer: 'her husband has completely lost his pillar of support and can be said to be utterly destituted'.

Far less sympathetic was *Native Opinion*'s Marathi obituary in its editorial, under the caption 'The Untimely Death of the Late Dr Mrs Anandibai Joshee'. It did not denigrate Indian women's foreign education outright, though it did drive the point home by stressing the allegedly supportive Gopalrao's presence in America and by briefly touching on Pandita Ramabai as a deterrent example of foreign travel. Her motto was stressed: 'I leave for America as a Hindu woman and I will return to this country as a Hindu woman'.

Very surprisingly, Mumbai's reformist *Indu-Prakash* published a rather casual obituary, not very sympathetic to women's education, in its Marathi column, 'Letters from Correspondents'. It alleged that only a few educated people mourned her death as a loss to the nation, but the common people knew nothing about her. 'She had accepted a challenge and exertion quite contrary to her physique and nature, she lived in a totally alien society, and acquired a difficult but useful science'. But her dreams and expectations were shattered just at the point of their fulfilment.

Predictably, dissenting voices were raised in order to undermine Anandibai's achievement. Soon after her death, the Marathi scandal sheet, *Pune Vaibhav*, which championed the conservatives' claim that she had not received a medical degree at all. *Kesari* (22 March 1887) took up cudgels on her behalf and confirmed that Anandibai did indeed earn the degree of doctor of medicine. *Pune Vaibhav* continued its attack, ridiculing the proposal of writing Anandibai's biography. This time the Marathi section of *Native Opinion* came to her defence:

The editors of the Vaibhav pose to those, who are engaged in writing the biography of the late Mrs Anandibai Joshee, the question: 'What is the life of this twenty-year-old lass, and what can one possibly write about it?' We do not understand why . . . [they] are so displeased with this woman. The poet

Keats died at about the same age, but his biography has been written, so can this woman's be written.

Kesari continued to keep Anandibai's memory alive in Maharashtrian hearts. It soon publshed the news (5 April 1887) that two of Anandibai's photos, her graduation photo taken in the United States and the one taken after her death, were available in a certain new photo studio. It suggested that her sympathisers should buy at least one of them and could get it enlarged and framed.

*

Anandibai's death had devastated Gopalrao, as testified by all the newspaper reports. When her ashes were collected, he did not immerse them in a holy river as was customary. 'With some difficulty and against the wishes of his people', wrote Mrs Dall, 'but doubtless with a strong desire to bear witness to Anandabai's devotion to this country', he sent them in a box to America, to be buried by the Carpenters in their family lot in the cemetery at Poughkeepsie, New York.[6]

Some time later he wrote to the Carpenters:

> I have given the contents of Dr Joshee's boxes to an English school, the founder of which Dr Joshee greatly admired.[7] They are arranged in a nice glass case and I hope they will be better cared for than they could be by me. It was a painful thing to see them all again.[8]

Thus ended the most meaningful chapter in Gopalrao's life. The mutual devotion of the couple had become legendary in contemporary Maharashtra, as had Gopalrao's – perceived rather than real – role in moulding Anandibai's personality and boosting her career. Anandibai's two biographers adopted very different stances vis-à-vis Gopalrao. In a typically Indian fashion, Kashibai Kanitkar, who knew him personally but only after Anandibai's death, gave him the credit for Anandibai's achievement – as did Anandibai herelf – and justified his whimsical and eccentric behaviour by reading a laudable ulterior motive in it. With Dall the case was otherwise: Gopalrao had given her reason to fulminate against him. Having seen him at close quarters in America and the effect his presence had on Anandibai, she was under no such compulsion and barely stopped short of condemning him outright, admitting that she wrote about him against her will: 'I have been obliged to allude to the conduct and published writings of Gopal Vinayak Joshee because they were involved in the history of his wife. I have done it as lightly and as briefly as possible'.[9] She also alleged that Gopalrao 'kept a steady eye to the advantages to be gained by Anandibai's thorough education' and tried to enlist the cooperation of missionaries in India under a false pretext. Dall's most telling comment is that 'those who heard him speak in this country will hardly understand the letter' addressed to the missionaries of Kolhapur in 1878.[10] These barely disguised charges of duplicity and untrustworthiness were founded on a ground more solid than Dall's admitted prejudice against Hindu men.[11]

Gopalrao's subsequent life was less illustrious and earned him notoriety rather than fame, though he kept himself in the limelight a few years longer. As in the case of Othello, Gopalrao's 'occupation was gone' with the loss of Anandibai, and he seems to have given up even the pretext of being a reformer. Uncurbed by Anandibai's restraining influence, he embarked on a series of pranks which were nothing short of obnoxious, enjoying the tacit support of Pune's conservative faction, whose overall leadership was claimed by Tilak and which was engaged in an increasingly acrimonious tussle with the reformers led by Ranade as well as Agarkar after his split with Tilak in 1888.

Initially Gopalrao lived on his fame as Anandibai's husband, a 'practising' rather than merely 'preaching' reformer who had proven the courage of his conviction, and a world traveller. In mid May 1887 he gave a talk on his 'Experiences of America' at the annual summer lecture series in Pune.[12] He then tried to consolidate his position among the anti-reform elite of Pune. An important part of their strategy for stalling social reform was to discredit the reformers and expose their alleged hypocrisy; in this effort Gopalrao served as a valuable tool.

His first initiative was to organise a tea party at St Mary's Convent (run by the Anglican 'Community of St Mary the Virgin') under the auspices of the Sisters. This was attended by a number of prominent local citizens, over fifty men and a dozen women. The event occurred on 14 November 1890, and a few months later Gopalrao published in *Pune Vaibhav* the entire list of guests, who included ideological adversaries Ranade and Tilak. Gopalrao claimed that they had drunk tea and eaten bisuits served by the missionaries and thus broken caste rules of diet for which they should be penalised, because the Pune elite were subject to the same caste norms as everybody else.[13]

The orthodox society of Pune unanimously clamoured for the ritual expiation of the alleged tea-drinkers. A select committee was instituted by the Hindu priests and laity of Pune to inquire into the matter, which came to be known as the 'Poona ostracism affair' (*gramanya*), or 'Panch Houd Mission Tea Party', the Anglican mission being located close to the convent. The inquiry commission was headed by representatives of Shankaracharya, and in its report, the *Mahratta* (5 July 1891) demanded that 'equal justice be meted out to all' and that 'this subject of the purity of the religion in hand' be treated seriously. None of the women had drunk tea at the party, and some of the men also confessed before the inquiry commission to having abstained. The remaining forty-two men – some of whom, like Ranade, had not drunk tea but refused to admit it for reasons of solidarity – were ostracised for almost two years. In the end Ranade consented to undergo purification, again out of solidarity with those who wanted a way out of the ostracism.[14] Tilak perfomed expiation at Banaras and wrote in *Kesari* in February to March of 1892 that the inquiry was a form of harassment because the only solid proof was with Gopalrao Joshee, who was not called as a witness by the orhodox faction for fear that he would embarrass them through unwanted exposés.[15] It is a measure of Gopalrao's nuisance value that he escaped personal retaliation or even criticism although he had implicated his allies, like Tilak, in the unsavoury incident.

Another of his pranks was the organising of a ceremonial wedding of a male and a female donkey on 18 December 1890 in collaboration with Vasudev Ganesh Joshi of the Sarvajanik Sabha (and known also as Vasukaka, or Sarvajanik Kaka). This was allegedly a comment on the reformers' futile attempt to stop old widowers from marrying prepubertal girls. The ceremony was well-planned, printed invitation cards were distributed, and the 'bridal pair' was paraded in a procession through the city streets.[16]

In February 1891 the Age of Consent controversy had reached its boiling point, and a pro-legislation meeting in Pune was attacked by a mob of students led by Gopalrao, among others.[17] Incidentally, the Bill was passed by the Supreme Legislative Council on 19 March 1891 and caused another outburst of protest. On 25 March 1891, *Shimga* (the day after Holi) was celebrated not only with the customary vulgarities but with the additional spectacle of 'a reformer's funeral', in which a sawdust-filled corpse, cheroot in mouth, biscuits in hand, and a liquor bottle on its chest, additonally adorned by broomsticks and old shoes, was carried in a procession past the houses of reformers, including that of the absent Agarkar, amidst a profusion of obscenities and slander. The procession was crowded with youngsters, but led by Gopalrao.[18]

Gopalrao's penchant for character assassination took other forms as well. He wrote a personal letter to Agarkar (who had condoled with him so warmly on Anandibai' death), hurling immoral accusations. Agarkar published an open letter addressed to him and his other critics in the Pune liberal weekly *Dnyan Prakash*, which soon published Gopalrao's apology as well.[19]

But Gopalrao's crowning sensation of these years was his sudden conversion to Christianity. On 29 June 1891 he was 'baptised and admitted into the Christian faith' by the Reverend Mr Taylor in a public ceremony at the famous spot known as the *Sangam*, the confluence of Pune's two rivers, as reported by the *Mahratta* 5 July 1891. The paper now took serious note of the lecture Gopalrao had delivered at several places in 1888 and 1889 on 'Hindu Social and Religious Reform'. This was basically a sketchy overview of his understanding of the evolution of Hinduism and of protest/reform movements over the centuries, as well as the persistence of the caste system. It was reproduced by the *Mahratta* in three instalments (2, 19, and 26 July 1891). Very cannily, Gopalrao kept one foot in the Hindu Brahmin camp even after his 'conversion' by continuing to wear his sacred thread and the sandalwood caste mark on his forehead. The somewhat predictable culmination of all this was his equally well-publicised and sensational 'reconversion' after about forty days, claiming that he had never ceased to be a Hindu Brahmin. Through all this spectacle, the *Mahratta* (which had mounted a strong attack on Ramabai after her conversion) as well as Pune Brahmins continued to treat him indulgently.

One more mischief he played during his period of 'conversion' was the news published in *Pune Vaibhav* (and perhaps planted by him) that he was planning to marry Pandita Ramabai, who had returned to India in early 1889.

In 1892 Gopalrao made a short and unsuccessful trip to England as a trader in Indian handicrafts, and published a Marathi travel account with a rather unbalanced commentary.[20]

He spent the last thirty years of his life at Nashik, staying intermittently with his brother's widow and his daughter Sai. On 8 October 1922 he died at Nashik, penniless, without family or friends. His sporadic notoriety notwithstanding, he left no mark on the social scene of Maharashtra, and remains best known as Anandibai's husband. His only other lasting contribution was the education of his niece Sai, later married to Wrangler R. P. Paranjpye of Pune.[21]

*

For a while after Anandibai's death, Gopalrao continued to keep in touch with the Carpenters. Not much is known of their subsequent lives, except that the family faced another tragedy in the death of twenty-eight-year-old Eighmie in 1899. She had been a school teacher at the time.[22] Her body was interred at the Poughkeepsie Rural Cemetery. Helena married William John Cobb of Walton, New York, on 15 August 1900, and the couple left for Colorado.[23]

In 1905 Mrs Carpenter is known to have corresponded with Dr and Mrs Satthianadhan of Madras. She also contribued an article on Anandibai which was published in *Indian Ladies' Magazine* in 1906. She died in March 1920 and was interred in the Poughkeepise Rural Cemetery. Mr Benjamin Carpenter then migrated to Colorado to join his married daughter Helena.

Helena Carpenter Cobbs' two childen, both sons, returned to New Jersey, where most of their children and grandchildren live.

Notes

1 The allusion is the poem by Keats, who also suffered from consumption.
2 The *Mahratta* was published on Mondays, but the issue of 28 March 1887 is not available.
3 My translation.
4 My translation. The editorial is credited to Agarkar by Y.D. Phadke: *Agarkara*, Mauja Prakasana Grha 1996, p. 156.
5 Cited in Bodley, p. v.
6 Dall, p. ix.
7 Possibly Victoria School run by Mr and Mrs Sorabji.
8 Dall, p. v.
9 Ibid, p. iv.
10 Ibid, pp. 32–33.
11 Ibid, p. 34.
12 *Kesari*, 10 May 1887.
13 R. Ranade, pp. 193–94; *Mahratta*, 5 July 1890.
14 R. Ranade, pp. 195–207.
15 Tilak, pp. 100–8.
16 Dhond, pp. 47; Phadke, p. 156.
17 Phadke, pp. 149–50.
18 Ibid, pp. 151–52.
19 Ibid, pp. 156–62.
20 Vaidya, 'Trishanku', in *Sankraman*, Pune: Shrividya Prakashan, 1985, pp. 70–95.
21 Saibai was the mother of Shakuntalabai Paranjpye and grandmother of the well-known playwright and filmmaker Sai Paranjpye.
22 *Elizabeth Daily Journal*, 18 October 1899.
23 Ibid, 16 August 1899.

REFERENCES

Agarkar, Gopal Ganesh. 1984. *Agarkar – Vangmaya,* edited by M.G. Natu and D.Y. Deshpande. Vol. l. Bombay: Maharashtra State Board of Literature and Culture.

Apte, H.N. 1929. *Haribhaunchi Patre* [Letters of Haribhau Apte]. Satara: Aikya – Sampadan Mandal.

Athavale, Parvatibai. 1928 (reprint, 2013). Mazee Kahanee. Pune: Rajhans Prakashan.

Balfour, Margaret I. and Young, Ruth. 1929. *The Work of Medical Women in India.* New York: Oxford University Press.

Bodley, Rachel L. 1981 (1887). "Introduction" in *The High-Caste Hindu Woman,* by Pandita Ramabai. Bombay: Maharashtra State Board for Literature and Culture. Reprinted.

Chakravarti, Uma. 1989. "Whatever Happened to the Vedic Dasi?" in *Recasting Women" Essays in Colonial History,* edited by Kumkum Sangari and Sudesh Vaid. New Delhi: Kali_for Women.

Chapman, E. F. 1984 (reprint). *Notable Indian Women of the 19th Century,* Inter-India Publications.

Chapman, E. F. 1891. *Sketches of Some Distinguished Indian Women.* W.H. Allen.

Conway, Jill Ker, ed. 1992. *Written by Herself: Autobiographies of American Women: An Anthology.* New York: Vintage Books.

Croasdale, Hannah T. 1888. "Tribute from the Faculty of Woman's Medical College of Pennsylvania" in *In Memoriam,* edited by Rachei L. Bodley, pp. 5–11. Archives of the Medical College of Pennsylvania.

Dall, Carolyn Healey. 1888. *The Life of Dr. Anandabai Joshee, a Kinswoman of Pandita Ramabai.* Boston: Robert Brothers.

Dhond, M.V. 1994. "Anandi Gopal" in *Jalyatil Chandra.* Pune: Rajahans Prakashan.

Guide to Collections in the Archives and Special Collections on Women in Medicine. MCP Archives.

Hartshorne, Henry. 1888. "Professional Tribute" in *In Memoriam,* edited by Rachel L. Bodley, pp. 20–22. Archives of the Medical College of Pennsylvania.

Heimsath, Charles H. 1962. "The Origin and Enactment of the Indian Age of Consent Bill, 1891". *The Journal of Asian Studies,* Vol. XXI, No. 4 (August), pp. 491–504.

———. 1964. *Indian. Nationalism and Hindu Social, Reform.* Princeton, NJ: Princeton University Press.

Hewat, Elizabeth G.K. 1953. *Christ and Western India.* 2nd ed. Bombay: Wilson College.

Joshi, S.J. 1970 (1968). *Anandi Gopal.* 2nd ed. Bombay: Majestic Book Stall.

————. 1996. *Anandi Gopal,* abridged translation from the Marathi by Asha Damle. Calcutta: Stree.

Joshi, Yashodabai. 1985 (1965). *Amcha Jeevan – pravas.* Reprint. Pune: Venus Prakashan.

Kanitkar, Kashibai. 1912. *Pa Va Sou Dr Anandibai Joshes Yanche Charitra va Patre* [Life and Letters of the Late Mrs. Anandibai Joshee]. Bombay: Manoranjan Grantha – prasarak Mandali.

————. 2002. *Dr. Anandibai Joshi Yanche Charitra* (Marathi Biography). 3rd ed. Ed. Anjali Kirtane. Mumbai: Popular Prakashan.

Karve, Anandibai. 1944. *Maze Puran,* edited by Kaveri Karve. Bombay: Keshav Bhikaji Dhavale.

Karve, Dhondo Keshav. 1928 *Atmavritta.* Hingne.

Keer, Dhananjay. 2017. *Mahatma Jyotirao Phule.* Mumbai: Popular Prakashan.

Kirtane, Anjali. 1997. *Dr. Anandibai Joshee: Kaal ani Kartritva.* Mumbai: Majestic Prakashan.

Kosambi, Meera, 1988. "Women, Emancipation and Equality: Pandita Ramabai's Contribution to the Women's Cause". *Economic & Political Weekly*, Vol. XXIII, No. 44 (29 Oct., Review of Women Studies). pp. WS 38–49.

————. 1991. "Girl-Brides and Socio-Legal Change: The Age of Consent Bill (1891) Controversy". *Economic & Political Weekly*, Vol. XXVI, Nos. 31 & 32 (3–10 August), pp. 1857–68.

————. 1992, "An Indian Response to Christianity, Church and Colonialisms the Case of Pandita Ramabai". *Economic & Political Weekly*, Vol. XXVII, Nos. 43 & 44 (24–31 Oct., Review of Women Studies), pp. WS 61–71.

————. 1994. "The Meeting of the Twain: The Cultural Confrontation of Three Women in Nineteenth Century Maharashtra". *Indian Journal of Gender Studies*, Vol. 1, No. 1 (Jan. – Jun.), pp. 1–22.

————. 1995a. *Pandita Ramabai's Feminist and Christian Coversions: Focus on Stree – Dharma Neeti.* Bombay: Research Centre for Women's Studies, SNDT Women's University.

————. 1995b. "Gender Reform and Competing State Controls over Women: The Rakhmabai Case (1884 – 88). Contributions to Indian Sociology.

————. 1995c. "The Politics and Premises of Gender Reform in Nineteenth Century Maharashtra" (Paper presented at the Seminar on Forms of Modern Consciousness in India: 19th and 20th Century, held at Chandigarh in January 1995. Forthcoming).

————. 1995d. "The Home as Social Universe: An Analysis of Women's Personal Narratives in Nineteenth Century Maharashtra" (Paper presented at the Sixth International Conference on Maharashtra: Culture & Society, held at Moscow, May 1995. Forthcoming).

————. 1996. "Dr. Anandibai. . . . . . .Image". *Economic & Political Weekly*, Vol. XXXI, No. 49 (Dec. 7).

————. 2007. "A Prismatic Presence: Anandibai Joshee Through Iconized Readings" in Crossing Thresholds: Feminist Essays in Social History, Ranikhet, Permanent Black.

———. 1999. "Realities and Reflections: Personal Narratives of Two Women from Nineteenth-Century Maharashtra" in *From Myth to Markets: Essays on Gender*, edited by Kumkum Sangari and Uma Chakravarti. New Delhi: Manohar Publishers and Distributors, pp. 125–160.

———. 2000. *Pandita Ramabai in Her Own Words*. Delhi: Oxford University Press.

———. 2016. *Pandita Ramabai: Life and Landmark Writings*. London & New York: South Asia Edition: Routledge.

Lerner, Gerda, ed. 1992. *The Female Experience: An American Documentary*. New York: Oxford University Press.

Lederle, M.R. 1976. *Philosophical Trends in Modern Maharashtra*. Bombay: Popular Prakashan.

Mayo, Katherine. 1927. *Mother India*. New York: Harcourt, Brace & Co.

Mies, Maria. 1980. *Indian Women and Patriarchy*. New Delhi: Concept Publishing Co.

Phadke, Y.D. 1996. *Agarkara*. Mauja Prakasana Grha.

Ramabai, Pandita. 1967 (1882). *Stri Dharma Niti*. 3rd ed. Kedgaon: Pandita Ramabai Mukti Mission.

———. 1981 (1887). *The High – Caste Hindu Woman*. Bombay: Maharashtra State Board for Literature & Culture. Reprinted.

———. 1889. *United Stateschi Lokasthiti. ani Pravasa – vritta*. Bombay.

———. 1977. *The Letters and Correspondence of Pandita Ramabai*, edited by A. B Shah. Bombay: Maharashtra State Board for Literature and Culture.

———. 1988. *Pandita Ramabai. yancha Englandcha Pravas*, edited by D.G. Vaidya. Bombay: Maharashtra State Board for Literaure & Culture. Reprinted.

Ranade, Ramabai. 1910. *Amchya Ayushyatil Kahi Athavani*. Pune: Dnyanprakash Press.

Said, Edward W. 1978. *Orientalism*. New York: Pantheon Books.

Sangari, Kumkum and Chakravarti, Uma. eds. 1999. *Myth to Markets: Essays on Gender*. New Delhi: Manohar Publishers and Distributors.

Scharlieb, Mary. 1929. "Foreword" in *The Work of Medical Women in India*, edited by Balfour and Young.

Stanley, Liz. 1987. "Biography as Microscope or Kaleidoscope? The Case of 'Power' in Hannah Cullwick's Relationship with Arthur Munby". *Women's Studies International Forum*, Vol. 10, No. 1, pp. 19–31.

Tilak, Bal Gangadhar. 1976. *Samagra Lokamanya Tilak*. Vol. V. Pune.

Tilak, Laxmibai. 1973. *Sampurna Smriti – Chitre*, edited by A. D. Tilak. Nasik.

Vaidya, Sarojini. 1985. "Trishanku" in *Sankraman*. Pune: Shreevidya Prakashan.

———. 1991 (1980). *Shreemati Kashibai Kanitkar: Atmacharitra ani Charitra*. [Mrs. Kashibai Kanitkar: Autobiography and Biography]. 2nd ed. Bombay: Popular Prakashan.

Varde, Mohini. 1991 (1982). *Rakhmabai: Ek Arta*. Bombay: Popular Prakashan.

Winslow, J.C. 1923. *Narayan Vaman Tilak: The Christian Poet of Maharashtra*. Calcutta: Association Press (Builders of Modern India Series).

* * * * *

Newspapers/ Periodicals:

Indian:

The Indian Ladies Magazine. Madras. 1906.
The Indu - Prakash [Anglo - Marathi weekly]. Bombay. 1883–1887.
The Kesari [Marathi weekly]. Pune. 1883 - 1912.
The Mahratta [English weekly]. Pune. 1883 - 1912.
The Native Opinion [Anglo - Marathi weekly]. Bombay. 1883–1837.
The Theosophis [English Monthly]. Calcutta and Madras. 1883–1887.
Vividha Dnyana Vistar [Marathi monthly].

American:

Frank Leslie's Illustrated Newspaper [Weekly]. New York, NY. 1883.
The Index [Daily]. Boston, MA.
The Philadelphia Evening Bulletin [Daily]. Philadelphia, PA. 1883. 1886.
The Philadelphia Inquirer [Daily]. Philadelphia, PA. 1883.
The Philadelphia Press [Daily]. Philadelphia, PA. 1886.
The Philadelphia Record [Daily]. Philadeplhia, PA. 1886.
The Missionary Review [Annual]. Princeton, NJ. 1878.

* * * * *

INDEX

Note: Page numbers in *italics* indicate figures. Page numbers that begin with P (e.g., P 01) indicate plates (located after p. 240). Page numbers that include an n indicate footnotes.

245

dominance of husband in 58–59; and
education of women 51, 69; European
vs. Indian 202; and *garbhadhan*
(impregnation) ceremony 19; Indians'
ideas about 43; married names
27n6; *see also* child marriage; Joshee,
Anandibai, marriage; Joshee, Gopalrao
Vinayak (husband); remarriage of
widows; widows
Mayo, Katherine, childbirth practices in
India 182
medical education 3; Anadibai's defence
of 91–92; Anandibai's early interest
in 41–42, 47; internship in Boston
185; need for women doctors in India
91–92, 145, 148–149; Ramabai,
Pandita and 92–93
missionaries 21–24, 35–36, 104
Missionary Review, The, Gopalrao's
letter about Anandibai's education 3,
29, 31
Mrs. Carpenter *see* Carpenter,
Theodocia

nationalism 84, 91–92, 161; Anandibai
and 48, 80, 89, 171, 173, 190;
cultural nationalism 181–182; and
social obligation 185; Anandibai's
speech on travel to U.S. 4; use of to
appeal to women doctors 92; *Kesari*
(Pune newspaper) 197; Ramabai,
Pandita and 161
New England Hospital for Women and
Children (Boston) 198; internship at
185, 198

obstetrics: Anandibai's thesis on
181–184; conditions in India 182;
see also women's health; medical
education
occult 64, 68; Anandibai's visions 5,
13, 74, 138, 143; Madame Blavatsky
48; Mrs. Carpenter and 5, 74; and
theosophy 48; *see also Theosophist, The*

Pandit, Vishnushastri, pioneer of widow
remarriage movement 16
Philadelphia, weather in 139–140,
142–143

Poughkeepsie (N.Y.) Rural Cemetery,
grave marker 1, *2*
Pune 11, 24, 91; Anandibai's cremation
at 3; Anandibai's death 228;
Anandibai's final illness 218–219,
222–223; Gopalrao's later life in
237–239; *see also* Joshee, Anandibai,
final illness

Ramabai, Pandita 54, 91–94, 104,
129–136, 139, 162, 196, 216,
218–19, 234–235, 235; Anandibai's
admiration for 3; comparisons
with Anandibai 92, 117, 130–131;
conversion to Christianity 117,
131–134, 148, 161, 196, 239; and her
physical appearance 192–193, 195;
husband's death 82; need for women
doctors in India 92–93; press coverage
of speech 195–196; *Stri Dharma Niti*
(book) 62; travel to England 137; visit
to U.S. 190–197, 205–207
rites 47; Anandibai's practice of 129,
131; at Brahmo Samaj wedding 80;
Mrs. Carpenter's interest in 41; of
passage 17–18; *see also* correspondence
with Mrs. Carpenter

sari *see* clothing, sari
Serampore 75–76

Theosophist, The 5, 125; Anandibai's first
letter to Gopalrao published in 6
travel to U.S.: Anandibai's 84–89; outcry
against Anandai's 91

widows 195–196; remarriage of 13–14,
16, 27n14, 50, 57, 133; treatment
of in India 43–44, 50, 69; *see also*
marriage
WMCP *see* Woman's Medical College of
Pennsylvania (WMCP)
Woman's Medical College of
Pennsylvania (WMCP): Anandibai's
study at 3, 87–88, 119, 124–125,
127, 132, 134, 181, 195, 232;
Anandibai with medical degree *191;*
commencement 190; committee
report of Anandibai's death P

Snippets from Anandibai's life and letters

Sources: Courtesy of Legacy Center Archives & Special Collections, Drexel University College of Medicine, Philadelphia. http://drexel.edu/LegacyCenter

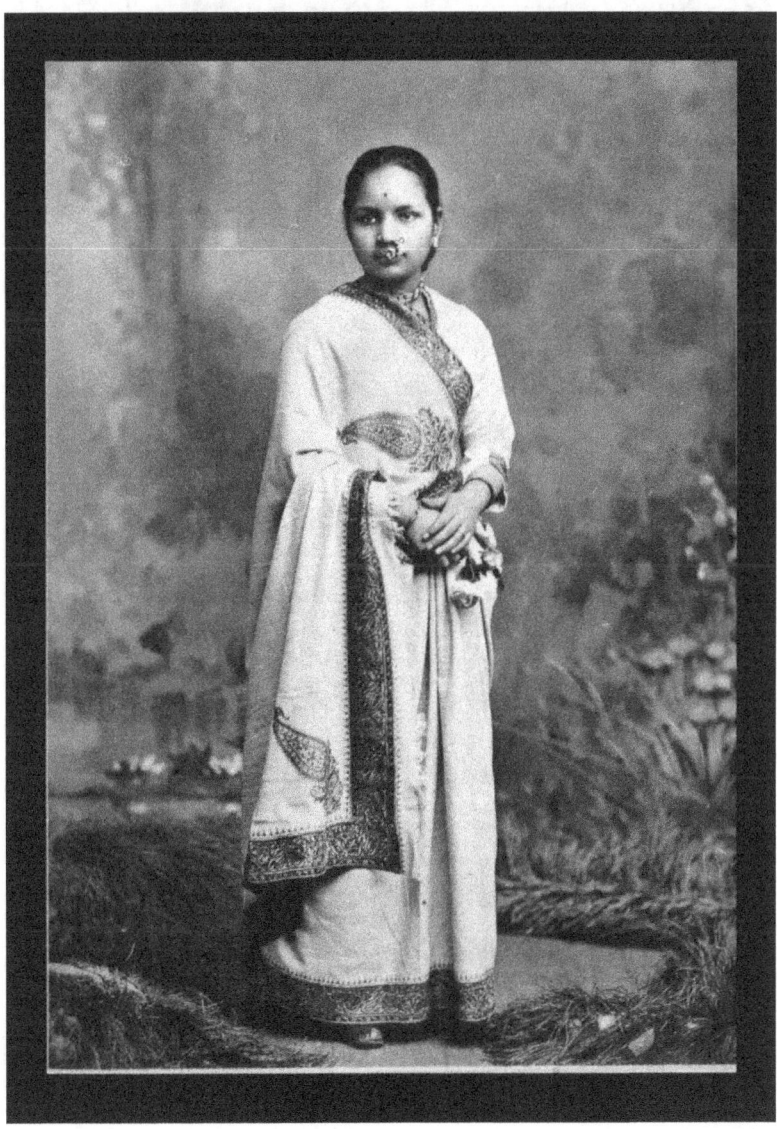

PUBLIC LEDGER

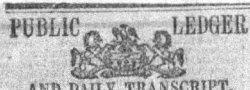

AND DAILY TRANSCRIPT.

Philadelphia, Tuesday, August 3, 1886.

BY THE QUEEN'S COMMAND.—The Queen of Great Britain and Empress of India, for many years holding opinions unfavorable to the recognition of medical women in her dominions, has yielded to the argument of accomplished facts. The Dean of the Woman's Medical College of Pennsylvania received last week from the Secretary of Legation of the United States (via Washington) a copy of a letter written at Windsor Castle, July 14, by the Queen's Private Secretary, General Sir Henry Ponsonby, addressed to Henry White, Secretary of the Legation, as follows: "I am commanded by the Queen to request that you will kindly thank Mrs. Bodley for having sent her Majesty the account of Dr. Joshee's reception in the Woman's Medical College of Pennsylvania, and to assure you that the Queen has read the paper with much interest." This recognition of Dr. Joshee, one of the Empress of India's subjects, by medical title is quite significant. Thanks to the eminent standing of the Woman's College here, and enlightened, perhaps, by the Vice Regent Lady Dufferin's warm interest in medical women in India sent out from this country, her Majesty is coming to the clearer understanding of the importance of this new title for a Hindoo subject.

THE FIRST WOMAN MEDICAL STUDENT FROM INDIA.

MRS. J. T. GRACEY.

As the Woman's Foreign Missionary society of the Methodist church was the first organization to send an educated medical woman to India, we believe it will be ready to extend a hearty welcome to the first medical student from that country as soon as she steps upon our shores. Mrs. Anadibai Joshee is a Brahmin lady of good social position, and comes here to enter the Woman's Medical college in Philadelphia for a thorough course of study. From a private letter we learn that she sailed from Calcutta on Monday, April 9, in company with Mrs. Dr. Lore and several missionaries returning to America, and is expected here early in June. Mrs. Joshee is young, only about nineteen, the wife of a Brahmin in the employ of the British government as postmaster at Serampore. He is a liberal-minded Hindoo, and in the hours he could spare from his business helped his wife in every way possible to secure what education she has, and now gives his full consent for her to come here and secure a medical training. The sacrifices this woman makes we here can scarcely appreciate. That she breaks away from all her associations, social and religious, to seek advantages in a land among strangers, and with a people so unlike her own in all their habits and customs, shows remarkable force of character. The step she takes is significant of the times, shows the breaking down of deep-seated prejudices, and is of peculiar importance. In coming, she must ignore the Brahmin creed, which prohibits them from crossing the water, eating food other than that prepared by Brahmins, or drinking water which has come in contact with other than vessels belonging to the caste, and many other restrictions, which involves the giving up of much that is so dear to a Hindoo. She does not come as a Christian woman, but from a benevolence of heart that seeks to help her unfortunate sisters. Before leaving her home she gave in the Serampore college a womanly address, explaining her reasons for her action, saying her great desire was to carry help to her own countrywomen. While in Calcutta, before sailing, she was the recipient of much kind attention, and we bespeak for her here, in this Christian land, the sympathy and affection of all women who have at heart the uplifting of woman in all countries.

(No 3.)

Union Co.

Roselle N.J. June 18th/83

Miss Rachel Bodley.
    Dear Madam,

        I have in my care Mrs Anandibai Joshee, a Hindoo lady of high caste. She has come to America to study medicine; that she might serve her fellow country women in the capacity of surgeon and physician. Hearing from many sources that the Female College of Pennsylvania is the best and most thorough in its main point, and believing from some things I have heard and seen in print that steps have already been taken to secure filthy

ward the advantages of your
College I write to ask you to
please inform me what
arrangements, if any, have
been made, also if Mrs Foster
would need to attend lectures
now before the close of this
term?

If she could begin her
studies at home with me,
and continue them through
the Summer, taking up such
as you deem necessary for
the beginning of a thorough
course, without incurring the
expense of a trip to Phila before
Fall, she would prefer to do so.
Her means are very limited
and the ways to obtain the
End in view is not yet clear.

We are in correspondence
with the Deans of several

Coll
plai
care
Bea
enr
had
in te
I fe
resp
your
whas
mad
adv
you
thou

et
bette
City, &
at he
Plea
and
frien

your Colleges, and shall form
plans for Mrs. Foster with
care and deliberation.

Believing that you or other
eminent Philadelphians
had already taken an interest
in her before her arrival, I
I feel willing and glad to
respect that interest by asking
your advice at the outset, and
what preparations if any have been
made for her and what her
advantages will be in
going to Philadelphia rather
than to New York?

It would suit our convenience
better to have her in the latter
city, but we have her best good
at heart, and seek only that.
Please find enclosed a letter
and circular from your
friend and ours, Mrs.

Reading M.O.
A reply at your earliest
convenience would greatly
oblige
Yours most respectfully
(Mrs.) Theodosia C. Carpenter

Miss.

Care
a Hi
She
stud
und
try
of s
Near
that
Penn
and
mea
from
Lea
that
been

[2291-00]

Woman's Medical College of Pennsylvania,

PHILADELPHIA, PA.

DEAN'S OFFICE, June 19th 1883.

Mr Alfred Jones,
Sec. of Ed. Committee,

Dear Sir:— This
morning's mail brings me
the first definite intelligence
I have rec'd, concerning the
arrival of Mrs Joshee, (the
Hindoo lady), in this country.

A half-dozen reporters of
the city press, representing as many
papers, have been calling
upon me and writing to me
in regard to her, during the
last month, so remarkable
do they regard her coming
to be.

I enclose the whole correspondence. The first letter will

Roselle N. J.
June 28th 1883

Alfred Jones Esqr
            Germantown,
                  Philadelphia, Pa.

Dear Sir,

            I beg to ask, if upon
any terms pecuniarily consistant
with my means, I may be allowed
to enter the Womens Medical College
of Pa. for a thorough course of study.
I have with me seventy dollars, and
my husband expects to send me
twenty dollars per month less the
cost of sending.

            I was eighteen years of age
last March.

            I have been once through
English Grammar, have studied
through Arithmetic in my own
language; & as far as Division in

English, and I am now pushing forward in this as fast as I can. I have read the histories of England, Rome, Greece and India.

I have learned to read and speak in Seven languages viz Marathi (my own) Sanscrit, Bengali, Gujarathi, Canari, Hindoostani, and English.

Though I may not meet in all points, the requirement for entering College, I trust, that as my case is exceptional and peculiar your people will be merciful & obliging. My health is good, and this with that determination which has brought me to your Country against the combined opposition of my friends & caste ought to go along way towards helping me to carry out the purpose for which I came viz to render to my poor suffering country women the true medi-

-cal aid they so sadly stand in need
of, and which they would rather die
for than accept at the hands of a male
physician. The voice of humanity is
with me and I must not fail. My
soul is moved to help the many who
can not help themselves, and I feel
sure that the God who has me in
his care will influence the many,
that can and should share in
this good work, to lend me such
aid and assistance as I may
need. I ask nothing for myself,
individually, but all that is
nessesary to fit me for my work
I humbly crave at the door of
your College, or any other that shall
give me admittance.

    For the kind encourage-
ment already recieved, and the
hopes held out, I feelingly subscribe myself, Yours gratefully,
Anandibai Joshee

Dec 9th 1887.

My dear friend,

In remembrance
of the beautiful life quickly
ended in Poona, India, in Feb.
1887, and which touched yours
in your College days, I wish to
call your attention to a remarkable portrait of our beloved
Dr. Joshee who is to be obtained
only in The High-Caste Hindu
Woman, a book written by her
cousin, Pundita Ramabai, and
issued in Philadelphia in June
1887. Facing the phototype is
a page In Memoriam, which
gives the important dates in
the brief life; in the Introduction
to the volume, I state all that
is definitely known in regard
to Dr. Joshee's death. The only
later intelligence that has been
received is, that some weeks
after the cremation of the body
the ashes were probably carried
to the distant Ganges, and cast

into its waters. Ramabai
still lives to carry on the
marvelous work of the elevation of Hindu women from
within their own ranks, so
unexpectedly laid down by the
brave little pioneer who could
claim our College as her alma
mater.

For several good reasons I am
very desirous that each class-mate
of Dr. Joshee shall own The High
Caste Hindu Woman, and I write
to request that if you do not already possess a copy, you will
purchase one at this Christmas
time and will if possible put it
upon your shopping list to purchase
as a gift for others, or will at
least induce some one to do this
in your stead. If Ramabai is
helped at all, she must be helped
at once and sent on her homeward
voyage, before our American climate begins its deadly work.

With kindest remembrances,
I am
Affectionately yours
Rachel L. Bodley.

[2291-609]

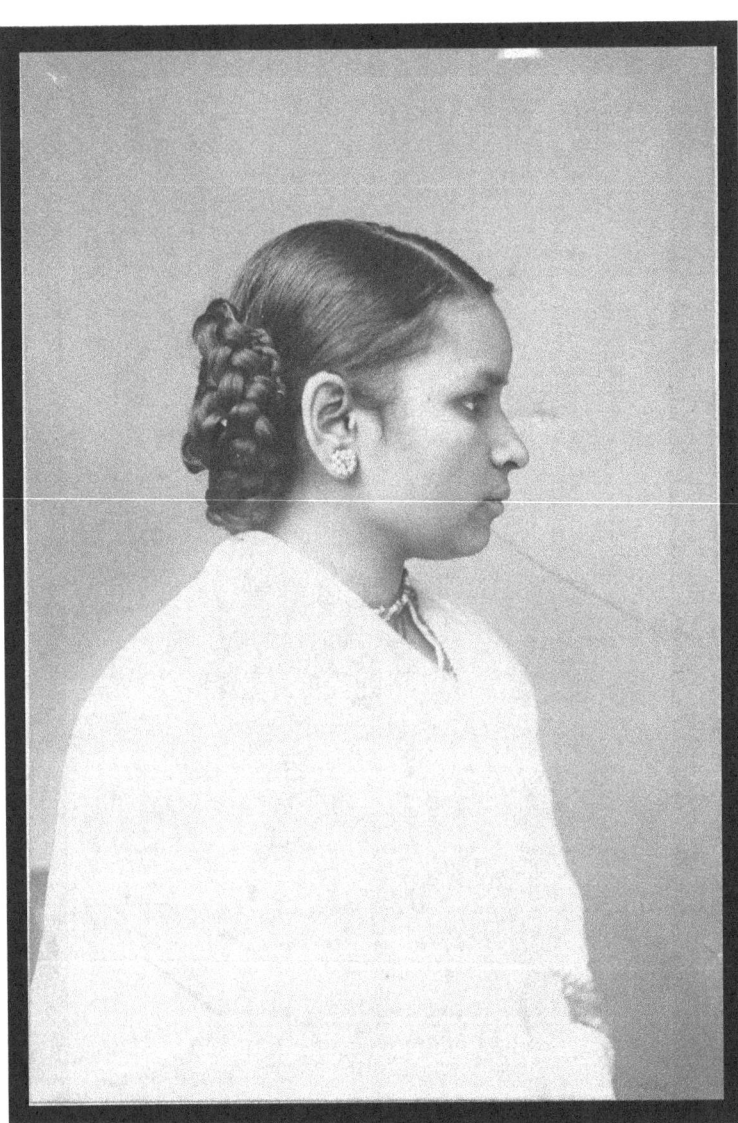

the corporators for this purpose is entirely inadequate to secure the constant services of a responsible librarian, and one has been here only at stated hours. There is no charge for the use of the Library. Through the summer months we have no librarian in charge, and the books can be seen through the chairman of the Library Committee, who will give an order to the janitor.

The report of the Committee on the Educational Fund was next in order, but the chairman of that committee not being able to reach Philadelphia on account of a severe snow storm, which prevented travel for several days, it did not arrive in time to be read at the meeting. It is as follows:

Report of Educational Committee.

Balance on hand March, 1887,	$207 90	
Received of Treasurer, 1887,	72 67	
		$280 57
Paid, Jan. 12, 1888, Prof. Hartwell for lectures on Physical Culture,	$60 00	
" Advertising Lectures,	7 20	
" Prof. Bodley for 100 Postal Cards,	1 00	
" " " Printing Postal Cards,	1 00	
		$ 69 20
Balance in Treasury March, 1888,		$211 37

E. C. KELLER,
Chairman of Committee.

The report of the Necrology Committee, which came next in order, did not arrive in time to be read at the meeting because of the storm. It is as follows:

Report of the Committee on Necrology.

DR. ANNA S. ADAMS (class of 1873) had a successful practice in Peoria, Ill., for thirteen years. She removed to Florida in 1886, where she died of pneumonia, October 25, 1887. Dr. Adams was twice sent as a delegate to the American Medical Association.

DR. ANANDIBAI JOSHEE, daughter of Ganpatrao Amritaswar and Gungbai Joshee. Born in Poona, Bombay Presidency, India, March 31, 1865. (Child name, Yamuna Joshee.) Married Gopalrao Vinayak Joshee, March 31, 1874. (Wife-name, Anandabai Joshee.) Sailed from Calcutta, India, for America, April 7, 1883, being the first high-caste Brahman woman to come to the United States. Landed in New York, June 4, 1883. Graduated in Medicine from the Woman's Medical

21

College of Pennsylvania, March 11, 1886, being the first Hindu woman to receive the degree of Doctor of Medicine in any country. Appointed June 1, 1886, to the position of Physician-in-Charge of the Female Ward of the Albert Edward Hospital, in the city of Kolhapur, India. Sailed from New York to assume her duties in Kolhapur, October 9, 1886. Died in Poona, India, February 26, 1887.

DR. GEORGIANA E. YOUNG (class of 1878) died at her home, Wesley Park, near Niagara Falls, October 23, 1887. She had long been in failing health, but while battling with disease had been courageously engaged in the practice of her profession.

DR. HARRIET BELCHER was born at Irvington, New Jersey, but at an early age removed with her family to Newark, N. J.

She was favored with excellent social and educational advantages, which were improved so far as her very delicate health would allow. Heavy care and responsibility came upon her while still a young girl, duties which were met by a judgment, self-reliance and executive ability, which marked her as possessed of great strength of character.

In 1875, the way opened for her to follow a long cherished desire to enter upon medical study preparatory to the life of a physician. She entered the Woman's Medical College of Pennsylvania in the autumn of 1875. Those who were associated with her can testify to her zeal and and faithful work as a student.

The Spring of 1877, she entered the New England Hospital for Women, in Boston, Mass., as interne; where she spent a year full of rich experience in her chosen profession, and won the high esteem of officers and patients. She returned to Philadelphia to attend the college session of 1878–9 and received her degree of M. D. in March, 1879. The same year she became a member of the "Rhode Island Medical Society." During 1878 and 1880 she responded a number of times to calls for public lectures upon subjects relating to hygiene and physical culture to audiences of women.

Her first settlement, in a conservative, prejudiced New England town, gave small promise for early success, and she wisely decided to seek a a better opening. In the winter of 1881 she looked for the last time upon loved and familiar faces, and alone crossed the continent to make for herself a home and friends among a strange people. Those who know how strong and tender were her attachments, how sweet the ties thus severed, can best appreciate the heroic courage and strength of will which held her firm to her purpose. At Santa Barbara, California, she found a field for faithful, earnest work, and attained an encouraging social and